Dearest 'Jenny,'
In celebration of you
and your adorable
step dog...
Here is Oscar's story!
With warm affection,
Jan Schwartz

with love
from Audrey

Last Summer with Oscar

An Adventurous True Story of Love and Courage

Jan Schwartz, Ph.D.

Last Summer with Oscar
An Adventurous True Story of Love and Courage
by Jan Schwartz, Ph.D.

Copyright © 2010 by Janet Mielke Schwartz
All rights reserved.
No part of this book may be reproduced in any form or by any electronic or mechanical means including information storage and retrieval systems without permission in writing from the publisher. The text, layout, and design presented in this book, as well as the book in its entirety, are protected by the copyright laws of the United States (17 U.S.C. 101 et seq.) and similar in other countries.

Fair use notice.
The use of the following media is protected by the Fair Use Clause of the US Copyright Act of 1976, which allows for the rebroadcast or republishing of copyrighted materials for the purposes of commentary, criticism and education.

One World Books
2550 Inverness Parkway, Northwest
Canton, Ohio 44708

ISBN: 9780983260127

Printed in the United States.
First printing August 2011. Second Printing December 2011. Third Printing August 2012.

*Dedicated to Oscar,
and all the beloved dogs in this world
who left us much too soon due to
cancer. We will remember what we
learned from you.*

*Dedicated to Winston,
and all of the beloved dogs who were
faithful companions to another "furry
one." We are heartened and hopeful
from your lessons of loyalty and
steadfastness, and ever so grateful for
the abundance of your grace.*

*Dedicated to Sugar,
and all of the beloved dogs who shared
time with us on the journey. Your
goodness enabled Light to shine even
when darkness entered the day.*

You live on forever in our hearts.

Table of Contents

Acknowledgments	**13**
A Note from the Author	**17**
Prologue	**21**
🐾 Chapter One: Last Summer With Oscar	**27**
The Diagnosis	27
Coming to Grips With Change	30
The Role of Attentiveness	33
Oscar Discovers Slippery Elm Leaves	38
The Catalog Arrives	47
Wingalings, Smothered Comfort and Working Dog's Stew	54
🐾 Chapter Two: Last Fall With Oscar	**63**
Cheering Him On!	63
Managing the Strain	70
The Leaves Fall Off	79
Gravizon From the Amazon	83
🐾 Chapter Three: Last Winter With Oscar	**89**
The Role of Fierce Pride	89
The Dark Surprise	91
Creative Feeding and the Community's Dog Food	100
Red Clover	106
The Heart Bowl	117
Our Effective Combination of Remedies	122

↬ Chapter Four: This Spring With Oscar — **131**
Watching the Remedies Work — 131
Smelling the Newly Budded Tree — 137
Love always, Oscar — 141

↬ Chapter Five: Epilogue — **149**
Winston's Response — 149
Dr. Heller's Response — 152
Dr. Pearson's Response — 153
Leaving a Legacy — 153

↬ Introduction to the Appendices — **157**
Appendix I: Slippery Elm and the Original Essiac Formula — 161
Appendix II: Only Natural Pet GI Support — 165
Appendix III: Only Natural Pet Immune Strengthener — 167
Appendix IV: PhytoPharmica Cellular Forté with IP-6 & Inositol — 171
Appendix V: NF Spectrum Probiotic — 175
Appendix VI: ONPS B.S.S.T. Herbal Formula — 179
Appendix VII: Oscar's Favorite Orange Chicken Recipe — 183
Appendix VIII: Gravizon — 187
Appendix IX: Red Clover — 189
Appendix X: Cellular Forte Max3 — 193

Acknowledgments

Writing a book of this nature requires time, quiet, detailed notes and great perseverance. Yet, after awhile, my spirit needed more. I found a secluded nook at the Arabica coffee house, and Laurel and Courtney Shaffer, two great dog lovers, provided me with unlimited kindnesses and the most gracious hospitality. During the final stretch of months spent writing *Last Summer with Oscar*, I surrounded myself with highly creative people, some old friends and some new, including successful writers and journalists, and many became my Facebook friends. I greatly admire the natural flow and cadence of your writing abilities, and feel privileged to count you among my friends. I also reconnected to some of my wonderful friends from Proviso West High School on Facebook. Know that your stimulating energy and our written conversations provided me with warm-hearted, delightful "breaks" in the writing of this challenging text.

Oscar's story was enriched by the suggestions offered by Mary Rhodes, Ginny Greenhill, Marcia Vahila, and Noelle Audi-Miller; the support of many police officers within the Hills and Dales Police Department and our friends and neighbors in the Village of Hills and Dales; the enormous caring of Dr. Charles Heller, and Joyce Carrick whose loving kindness furthered our hope of healing; Dr. Ben Pearson, for his compassion and encouragement; Anne Weiser, and her wonderful staff at the Orrville Pet Spa, for showing great love to Winston which nurtured the renewal of his joy; and, my dear and wonderful friends,

Congressman and Dr. Mary Regula, for their great belief and support. Bless you all for your most wonderful ways!

An abundance of gratitude is extended to my parents, siblings and extended family for all they have taught me, and for all we have learned together.

I remain grateful to Dr. Robert O'Block for his vision and guidance, to Marianne Schmid for her belief in my mission to promote the power of good, and to the gifted and talented ACFEI Media Team for their many professional kindnesses. I especially want to acknowledge Cary Bates, who made the publication process a truly wonderful experience.

And finally, to my husband, Richard, for his love and understanding in the writing of this book, for his joyful caring of Oscar, and for truly sharing in our miraculous lifelong journey.

A Note from the Author

It may be helpful for the reader to learn that Oscar and Winston were happy and healthy dogs who received consistent doses of love and attention, regular walks and plenty of exercise. Visits to the vet were primarily for routine check-ups, or for a sprained paw that resulted from their playful pursuits with each other or with other animals who visited them in our backyard. For many years they ate a very high quality dog food that I purchased at a pet store, but when weight loss became a necessity, they ate a vet-prescribed dog food. As with most golden's, they loved to eat, and received, perhaps, more than their share of treats! They lived in a pampered-dog household. They also loved having baths and certainly had plenty of them! Their paws were wiped off prior to entering the house especially when they partook of one of their favorite pastimes: digging in the mud.

Their paws were wiped off for other reasons, too. The products used on our lawn were chemicals administered by the crews that serviced our yard. Oscar and Winston were kept inside during the various lawn applications, and they remained inside until the application had dried. For days after the application of lawn treatment, we would wash off their paws with water, using fresh towels, when they had played on the grass. We also did not allow them to lick their paws following contact with freshly treated grass.

They were not permitted to walk on other lawns that had just been treated. Thankfully, the lawn crews always placed a notification sign on the neighborhood lawns when an application had been applied. Organic products were not an option for us at the time, but, in general, we thought we were doing nearly all we could to prevent cancer. I share these facts as dog lovers asked about these issues as I was writing the book. Most dog owners want to be certain they are doing all they can possibly do to keep their dog healthy.

All of the information and details mentioned in this book are true. It was very important to me to describe the incidents and experiences with great accuracy. I humbly offer this story with the sincere hope that I have honored the integrity of our cherished Oscar's and Winston's journey.

Jan Schwartz

Prologue

What is behavioral science? According to www.wisegeek.com, "behavioral science is a branch of the sciences which is concerned with the study of human and animal behavior. Behavioral science looks at individuals and their behaviors along with the behavior of societies, groups, and cultures, and processes which can contribute to specific behaviors...behavioral science tends to look at the reactions within and between organisms which dictate behavioral trends." The FBI Academy describes behavioral science as "all about better understanding criminals and terrorists—who they are, how they think, why they do what they do—as a means to help solve crimes and prevent attacks (www.fbi.gov/about-us/training/bsu)."

My work as a forensic behavioral scientist began 19 years ago when I discovered some evidence that catapulted me from developing a free family therapy clinic to a career in forensic fraud research. With great effort and unusual collaboration with state and federal authorities, the initial evidence unfolded into numerous state and multi-state investigations. This provided the impetus for future efforts in conducting forensic fraud research, performing white-collar organized crime investigations and facilitating other projects that worked to help strengthen our government.

Forensic Fraud Research, Inc., is a non-profit, not-for-fee investigative firm that formally incorporated in 2000, and became affiliated with the National White Collar Crime Center in 2003 (www.whitecollarcorruption.com). It is comprised of skilled professionals as well as state and federal employees who, together, aspire to the purpose listed on the incorporating papers. As president, I am the only face associated with the firm. All sources, whistleblowers and members within the network are kept confidential unless permission is granted for disclosure.

In 2005, the U.S. Department of Justice requested permission to videotape my presentation, "Psychology of White-Collar Criminals," for use on their Justice Television Network. Nineteen years of intelligence-gathering efforts and research while conducting semi-structured interviews with more than 250 victims, whistle-blowers, alleged offenders, offenders and alleged offenders' spouses and family members, witnesses and bystanders resulted in the identification of the "Behavioral Characteristics and Personality Traits of the White-Collar Organized Criminal and the White-Collar Organized Community."

In my career as a forensic behavioral scientist, it has been a privilege to compile data for and provide information to the HIDTA Money-Laundering Division of the FBI in Manhattan, the FBI in Washington, D.C., the Defense Intelligence Agency, the National Science Foundation, the Criminal Investigation Division of the IRS, the U.S. Department of Health and Human Services, the U.S. Postal Inspections Service, the Ohio Organized Crime Investigations Commission, the Ohio Attorney General's Office and 19 other state departments in addition to various United States Attorney's Offices. Writing "The Psychological Profile of a Spy (2006)" for the American Board for Certification in Homeland

Security, and conducting a pilot program for the nation, "Overcoming Resistance on the Local Level (2008)" are among the activities that blended my work into the fields of intelligence and homeland security.

However, in order to be able to write this book, some may wonder about my academic credentials. I received a B.S. in Education from Valparaiso University, and my M.Ed. and doctoral degrees from the University of Pittsburgh. At the University of Pittsburgh, I received the distinction of University Scholar, which is an award presented to "one of those who show high promise of significant contribution to society and progress." I also had the wonderful experience of completing a clinical research practicum at Western Psychiatric Institute and Clinic, the University of Pittsburgh School of Medicine, in the Children's Psychiatric Treatment Services Unit under Alan E. Kazdin, Ph.D.

It may also be helpful for the reader to know that I have been an Adjunct Professor of Behavioral Sciences at the Northeast Ohio Universities College of Medicine. I have also been Chair and Chair Emeritus of the American Board of Forensic Examiners. Presently, I am a member of the Executive Board of the American Board of Forensic Examiners. I am a fellow of the American College of Forensic Examiners, a diplomate of the American Board of Forensic Examiners (primary areas: family therapy, forensic fraud research and pain management), a diplomate of both the American Board of Forensic Medicine and the American Board of Psychological Specialties (triple boarded: behavioral science; family/marital/domestic relations psychology and medical psychology) as well as a diplomate of the American Academy of Pain Management. Further, I am Certified in Homeland Security Level V (CHS-V), and am a member of the Executive Advisory Board of the American Board for Certification in Homeland Security. I am an Intelligence Analyst, Certified (IAC), and also serve on the Executive Advisory Board of the American Board of Intelligence Analysts.

In February of 2011, I was appointed Chair of the International College of the Behavioral Sciences (www.behavioralsciences.org).

Now that I have told you what has come before, I am ready to share Oscar's story.

CHAPTER ONE

Last Summer With Oscar

✤ *The Diagnosis*

I grabbed my lavender sweater set thinking that the wonderful color might help to make me feel better. Dressing hurriedly, I focused on what I needed to accomplish before I joined Richard, my husband, in the car. I took several moments to hug Winston, Oscar's littermate, and reassured him as I snuggled his sweet face, saying that very soon Oscar would be home. It may sound unusual that the two dogs had never been apart, but they were, in fact, inseparable. By nature's own design, their life in our household was a shared and joyful experience.

But, change was in the air. Feelings of anticipatory grief muted the beauty of the spring day, and I struggled to keep my mind on task. We had dropped off Oscar, our 9-year-old much beloved Golden Retriever, at the Animal Care Clinic at 7 p.m. the evening before for tests and x-rays. And now, we were scheduled to meet with Dr. Heller at 9:30 this morning.

It seemed surreal that these moments were actually happening in real time, and not in a dream. Oscar was a formidable dog; he was effervescent, and quite unstoppable in his joy and zest for living. And yet, the events of the last months had seemingly worked to dampen the spirit of this nearly perfect dog. A torn due claw, normally such a routine happening, had turned into a botched and bungled nightmare due to the dysfunction and mismanagement of another pet care team. Now, two vets later, we placed the care of our adorable bundle of fur into the hands of a man who seemed to value animals as more than just a business opportunity. He knew of what we'd been through, and tried hard to convey his scientific knowledge with sensitivity in response to our questions regarding the fluctuations in Oscar's weight.

He'd regained the 9 pounds he had lost before we took a spring vacation to celebrate Richard's birthday. The trip had been a special present from me, and we returned home feeling refreshed and renewed. However, I knew something was wrong when I picked up the dogs from a well-respected boarding facility. *"Are you sure that everything went along OK, Joe?"* I asked as both Oscar and Winston leaped into the back seat of the car. Oscar's eyes flashed dark with fear, and their intensity had taken me by surprise. Joe paused, and then nodded his head rather unconvincingly.

But all was not well. Something was majorly wrong; both once hearty eaters, Winston munched in solo while Oscar anxiously paced in place while trying to force himself to eat. I made a point of being with them as they ate. Oscar could tell that I noticed the change, and kept looking up at me for help. Not wanting to alarm him any further, I began to play a food game to entice him to eat. But, by the second day of food games, Richard and I knew we had to act quickly, and Dr. Heller agreed. We needed to determine the cause of Oscar's behavior change.

It was the 10th of May, and as we drove off to the Animal Care Clinic in silence we did so with prayers and high hopes that, no matter what, all would again be well. Upon our arrival, the receptionist took us back immediately to the surgical area to meet with our new vet. Dr. Heller was not alone in the room. A special youngster had been "interning" with him that morning, and the precocious 7-year-old greeted us like a pro. He offered to keep Oscar "company" while we accompanied Dr. Heller to view the x-rays.

I glanced at Richard, who was especially close to this dog, and wondered if he, as a surgeon, already knew what we were about to hear. I could tell that he was bracing himself as well, and this brought tears to my eyes. This beautiful dog, this dog who had brought so much joy and goodness into our house! Please let the news be not so…

Dr. Heller spoke kindly but firmly as he pointed to the large tumor masses. While Oscar's CBC had been normal, the tumors were sizes of such significance that the vet felt our time left with Oscar was minimal. Richard asked him for a prognosis based on his extensive experience. "Sixty days," he said with a voice and manner that seemed to indicate two weeks. "Dogs with this cancer die from being unable to eat."

How could this dog of abounding joy and energy have only weeks to live? Our thoughts were reeling as he told us chemotherapy was now available for dogs, but that this was its own journey and process. It might prolong his life for 6-9 months. I looked at Richard, and knew that I spoke for us both: "Thank you, Dr. Heller, but no, we will not put Oscar through that. We would never want to do anything that could break his spirit." As the tears streamed down my cheeks, I managed to say, "We will celebrate this magnificent dog every single day we have left with him."

Dr. Heller seemed to be surprised by my response, but there was nothing more for any of us to say. Richard and I began to gather Oscar's things, and as we placed him on his leash the endearing young "intern" turned toward us and provided us with a tender and compassionate farewell. "He was the best-behaved dog here today!!" he exclaimed.

God, forever bless this child who so ably shares the gift of kindness.

Coming to Grips With Change

By the next afternoon, I knew that it would be impossible for me to sit by helplessly and allow Oscar to die one molecule at a time. "What can I do," was the mantra running endlessly through my mind, and my footsteps led me to visit with my good friend, Mary Rhodes, at the National First Ladies' Library. Mary was a devoted animal lover, and she had shared many a situation with me regarding her use of holistic remedies.

As she listened to me she did so with a keen understanding, and I felt glad that I had come by. This was my first experience with dog cancer, and I appreciated being able to share the facts with someone who had experienced this harsh reality. She saw that my channel of thought was temporarily blocked by acute sadness, and that I was stuck on our vet's undeniable conclusion. "Never lose hope, Jan," she said. "Everyone deserves to hope!" I was comforted in hearing this, and we began to discuss home-cooked foods that Oscar might be able and willing to eat.

In putting together a plan of action, I agreed that it would be a good beginning step to make a mixture of rice with drained, lean ground beef, with more ground beef than rice in the proportions. I stopped at the store and loaded up on the essentials, and returned home to immediately begin the plan.

It brings me joy in remembering the moment Oscar (and, of course, Winston, too) was presented with a small portion of the ground beef and rice. He got up from where he was lying down from the aroma, and after a few sniffs, eagerly began to eat, and in no time whatsoever, ate what I had placed before him. I sensed that he was *starved*, so I gave him another 10 oz. portion to see what would happen. He devoured the second, the third and, yes, even the fourth package of the food!

This time, Richard and I were both standing beside the dogs as they ate, and when Oscar finished the fourth package he looked up at us contentedly. Securely attached, he was capable of communicating his needs to us, and for this we were grateful. We did so want to provide him with what he needed, and pledged to each other that we would continue to search for the "right fit" of food to feed him throughout this journey. Our hearts were filled with hope.

Several days later Oscar finally had a bowel movement. By the fifth day another pet-loving friend commented that she couldn't believe how well he was doing. "He wasn't even able to hold his head up before, and look at him now!" Ginny said. She encouraged me to keep a log of everything we were doing for him. "A lot of people wouldn't know what to do if this happened to them, Jan." I looked at her, and realized that she meant it. From that point on, I made copious notes of all the "Oscar details."

Nine days later, Oscar was once again a happy dog! He was eating normally, and was his normal energetic self. He even begged for a walk! So it was on May 19th that Oscar and Winston *took me* for our customary three-mile walk in our hilly and wooded neighborhood.

But, two weeks later, Oscar appeared to be losing interest in the rice and beef. I read through some veterinary books I'd found in our groomer's library, and noted the recommendation of a high protein diet. The protein could be paired with bread, noodles or rice. Our dogs *loved* bread! In fact, breakfast for Richard all of these years had meant sharing his asiago bagel with Oscar and Winston, who devotedly sat on either side of him. The predictability of receiving a reward was more than highly likely, so they didn't move an inch and waited patiently for the piece or two that Richard faithfully gave them. Yes, we would try using bread, and we would also switch the protein whenever Oscar seemed to lose interest!

Years earlier, I had learned from a pet cookie baker that dogs loved the taste of tuna. That evening I experimented, and gave Oscar a whole can of tuna in water that I mixed with small pieces of a bagel. He loved it! On another day, we offered him brown rice with *chicken*, and he loved this so much that I found myself roasting up to nine whole chickens to produce enough protein for the week. His appetite was once again spectacular!

Oscar and Winston did everything as a team, and as they always ate together previously, we kept this pattern in place to maintain stability, to allow for a feeling of normalcy. (Our efforts to feed them separately had yielded much distress and confusion for the dogs.) Winston continued to eat his usual dog food, but he was also given a little rice mixture on top. Amazingly, he didn't appear to be stressed about Oscar receiving more. In observing them as they ate together, Winston seemed to understand that something was wrong with Oscar. But, then again, being intuitive, dogs just seem to "know" these things.

What Oscar and Winston also knew was that we adored them. They had so many precious ways of conveying their devotion to us as well. Thus, the cancer only intensified the strength of the bond between us.

The Role of Attentiveness

Noting significant milestones helped us to feel that we were making progress in the battle for wellness. However, it wasn't just eating habits that needed to be noted. We also began to track Oscar's body habits. Thankfully, and finally, a soft stool appeared on May 29th.

On June 2nd, we took our *fifth* three-mile walk. It had been a great day, but the surprise of diarrhea (which is a chronic issue with dog cancer) that evening posed a real challenge as Oscar would awaken suddenly, having a great need to go outside immediately. He did so several times that night. Obviously exhausted, he (and Winston) slept much of the next day. However, the aroma from two Amish chickens roasting seemingly enticed his appetite, and he was able to eat nearly an entire pound of chicken with the rice. Getting him to eat was, undoubtedly, Richard's and my top priority.

The sudden physical changes, the ups and downs of mood, the good days, bad days or parts thereof—caring for a family member or loved one with cancer requires a great flexibility of spirit and a focused attentiveness. A caregiver learns this one way or another, and the significant lesson was conveyed to me quite vividly in a dream.

In my dream, I was searching for Oscar in various locations with all sorts of imposing shapes and interferences impeding my search. I was beckoned high and low, and my concern grew stronger when he was not in any of the predictable places. I searched to the right and to the left, down this road and the next. I began to run as moments of time clicked away, and I searched harder and ran faster. It was then that I saw him. I sensed that time was running out. But, I couldn't get any closer to reach him, and had to lean over a walkway and stretch myself as far as was humanly possible to grab him to keep him from completely slipping through a crack in a steel-braced glass door. His dark, fearful eyes spoke volumes to me. I realized from the look on his face that he had been waiting for me the entire time of my search.

The next morning I sat quietly and pondered the meaning of the dream. I concluded that I needed to match wherever he was emotionally and physically. I needed to be in touch, in sync and attentive to everything, and needed to focus on bringing an integration of body, mind and spirit. Mopy? What helped him snap out of boredom before? What mischief or silliness would delight him? I also knew that I could never again bear to have him longing for my help without realizing it. And, neither could Richard.

June 4th brought us a big surprise—Oscar greeted us when we came home, and gave us his usual demanding bark for food!

June 5th was a day that required playing silly games with Oscar to encourage his eating. Today's game worked effectively. I gave him a whole large Milkbones cookie (always a favorite), and then took another half from the box as he eagerly watched. I stacked them on top of each other and presented him with both. His tail wagged slowly at first, unsure about the abundance of treats, and then more quickly as his entire body moved with joy at the silliness. He was surprised and delighted! Treats had never been given more than one at a time, and most certainly never presented to Oscar and Winston in this way. He enjoyed the game so much that the next day we gave him two stacked Milkbones, and he responded with much silliness in return.

June 9th brought increased hope as his stool was now formed... Oscar's body felt exceptionally warm, and he chose to sleep at night on the cool bathroom floor. Tonight, I began a new routine that I want to continue. Just before he went to sleep, I knelt beside Oscar, put my arms around him, and prayed out loud (I did the same with Winston). He seemed to be comforted by these humbly stated creations, and would let out a deep sigh as I began to pray aloud with great conviction. Tonight's prayer was: "Father God, with joy and thanksgiving I raise-up our beloved Oscar. You know his every need. Help us to know how to care for him. Please, Father God, heal his body, heal his heart and heal his spirit. Fill his body with Your all-healing Light. May he feel the warmth of your love surrounding him. We are grateful for the gift of this journey in our lives. Please grant us the strength, courage and ability to walk the path. To the glory of Your name! Amen."

June 10th: It is now one month from the date of Oscar's diagnosis. Oscar continues to do well, and he has resumed the role of "gamester" in our household. Much to our delight, he played the "watch me shred the Kleenex from the bathroom trash can" game today. This time, however, he was puzzled when we didn't correct him, but, rather, I cheered at his performance as we were given another opportunity to enjoy his mischief.

June 11th: Oscar ate one pound of drained, ground beef with brown rice in the morning. Amazing!

June 12th: More growths appear on his body, but his stool remains solid. We took our seventh three-mile walk.

June 13th: This was a very good day, and Oscar had a normal stool.

June 16th: While I am in Chicago, Oscar was not able to eat the ground beef with rice that I had prepared and left for Richard to give to him. To keep him eating, Richard brought home a plain Chick-fil-A sandwich. He cut-up the sandwich as Oscar watched, hoping to increase his appetite as the aroma was released. Richard told me he blew on each piece of the sandwich after he cut it to help it cool. Oscar received an abundance of Richard's love through these gestures, and he ate the sandwich in no time as a result. It is enormously gratifying to discover something that Oscar will eat! I understand that Oscar ate another plain Chick-fil-A sandwich at dinner. He loved it! (But, of course, Richard gave Winston a little sample both times as well.)

June 17th: Oscar just nibbled on the beef with rice mixture this morning, so we tried another protein and starch. I offered him tuna with wide egg noodles, but he was disinterested. Next, I warmed up two slices of garlic bread leftover from dinner, and put two cans of tuna in water on top. It was a hit, and he loved it! I decided to buy some honey wheat sandwich buns and dinner rolls at the grocery store today to try to keep Oscar interested. He seems anxious at meal time as he is eager to please us. It is best to have back-up food on hand at all times.

June 18th: Took our eighth three-mile walk today. All of our "doing" is helping us manage our feelings of helplessness. Oscar is acting much more secure today, and so is Winston.

Thankfully, we all seem to be doing better today.

✒ *Oscar Discovers Slippery Elm Leaves*

June 20th: Feeding Oscar canned tuna in water mixed with honey wheat rolls or honey wheat sandwich buns continues to work when he's experiencing diarrhea. Thank goodness! Oscar and Winston took me for our ninth three-mile walk.

June 21st: I stopped over at the Animal Care Clinic to buy another bag of prescription dog food and Rimadyl for Winston. The staff very gently inquired about Oscar, and seemed quite surprised at my answer. I told them Oscar is still alive, and is taking three-mile walks every other day with us!

June 24th: An employee at a local deli, suggested that I offer cottage cheese to Oscar. He was unable to eat until 10:30-11 a.m. this morning, and I needed to feed him by hand to create any interest in eating. I offered him cottage cheese at noon, but he was disinterested. I introduced the combination of lamb with rice in the p.m., and Oscar ate his entire dinner with gusto!

Oscar's discovery: This was an interesting evening. While on our tenth three-mile walk, Oscar suddenly lunged with great curiosity into a patch of natural brush, and, after actively sniffing in a cluster of bushes began to eat some of the leaves. At first, Winston just stood there watching Oscar chomp on the leaves, but then he barged in to join the fun. I kept an open mind and refrained from pulling them back on task. They were on an unmaintained piece of property along the road, and seemed to be having fun. Besides, with all of our walks and experiences, I had learned to trust that they would not eat or drink anything that was harmful to them.

June 26th: Our 11th three-mile walk. Interestingly, this was the second evening they wanted to stop to eat the special tree leaves. I decided to ponder privately about this, but couldn't help wondering if Oscar had discovered something significant.

June 27th: Unfortunately, Oscar was disinterested in the tuna mixture this morning. Having nothing else already prepared to feed him other than Winston's prescription diet dog food, I put one and a half cups of it in the bowl, and Oscar quickly ate it. What a surprise! I put more dog food in the bowl, but he walked away.

June 28th: This was an exceptionally beautiful summer day, and the dogs and I enjoyed the gentle breeze when we began our afternoon walk. Just as we were passing a neighbor's home, a branch from one of the old, established trees along the road swayed toward us, and Oscar jumped up to try to grab a leaf as it brushed over him. Did he smell something? I wondered. Keeping an attentive eye on him, I noticed that he looked back to connect his eyes with mine, and, remembering my dream, I paid close attention to this new behavior. What was he conveying to me? I looked carefully at the leaves so that I could identify them elsewhere. We continued on our walk, and I noticed that as we came down the hill and approached the unmaintained section of land where they discovered the leaves, Oscar and Winston's gait began to speed up. Sure enough! They more-or-less pulled me along with them into the brush, sniffed around, and began to eat the same leaves. This time, I was convinced that what was happening was relevant. I noticed they chewed on some leaves, but passed over others. My curiosity was piqued, and I decided to mention all of this to Richard that evening. When I conveyed all of the details to him, he nodded his head and listened thoughtfully, agreeing that this development was very interesting. He echoed my feelings, and encouraged me to learn more about the leaves.

June 30th: Today, we took our 13th three-mile walk. As we were again walking during daylight, I was determined to get a better look at the leaves while they were eating them. I noticed jagged edges on the leaves and also some tiny fibers; Oscar would chomp on some, but also would slide a leaf or two through his mouth. The same was true with Winston. How fascinating! They appeared to be energized from the experience, and I allowed Oscar to eat the leaves for as long as he wanted to. He seemed to have his own satiation point…Also, today, we introduced French toast to Oscar for his morning feeding, and made it with a wonderful Italian bread (Pane Turano) that I found at a small, family-owned store that featured foods grown on their farm and orchard. The French toast was a huge hit, and so was the evening meal of multi-grain bread (health food store) mixed with canned tuna in water.

July 1st: The lack of sleep is catching up with me, and I planned to head back to sleep after letting the dogs out early this morning. As tired as I was, I truly didn't mind it at all when Oscar banged the bedroom door open and burst in to wake me! It has been such a long time since I've awakened to his cold nose and wet kisses…We were low on tuna, so I made French toast again for Oscar's morning feeding…Both dogs came outside with me later, but before long I realized I had a little helper working beside me. Oscar "helped" with the pruning of the dead parts of the perennials by attempting to imitate what I was doing. He chomped off the black tips of the iris.' This is the second time he has "worked" with me in the garden!

July 2nd: Oscar was interested in having his vitamin and cookie along with Winston this morning! We also took our 14th three-mile walk.

July 3rd: This was the second day that Oscar ate his vitamin and cookie with Winston in the morning! It is so comforting to have another daily routine resume for us.

July 5th: At 7 a.m., Oscar vomited as he was walking down the stairs. Golden Retrievers are sensitive dogs, and we can tell these are embarrassing moments for him. He walked away as we cleaned up the mess and headed over to a favorite spot to rest peacefully...At 9 am, I offered him some French toast. He ate a few pieces and licked others fiercely, but then walked away. He rested and slept all day long...However, when I came home I found his favorite gorilla toy by the back door along with some pieces of shredded Kleenex from one of the small trash cans. He was just laying there in the family room watching me and waiting for me to react to his mischief. I was only too happy to nuzzle his sweet, beautiful face...Later on, he and Winston came over to me with both of their tails wagging, begging for a walk, but I was unsure about going for a walk as he had been so ill in the morning. I decided to go with the flow. As we were walking, it occurred to me that I didn't need to be concerned. *Both dogs simultaneously cut the walk short at the halfway point by turning down a street that led us back home.* Once again, I was reminded of their sixth sense and keen ability to communicate with each other.

July 7th: I picked up another bottle of Rimadyl for Winston from the vet's office and spoke at length with Joyce Carrick as she closed up the clinic. She was genuinely enthusiastic about Oscar's progress, and felt it was such a wonderful story. She suggested a healing might be taking place, and encouraged me to write about it to help others. Her kindness, and warm, caring words of support were so comforting...That evening, Oscar ate a mixture of asiago bagel with tuna, and asiago bagel with freshly roasted chicken. This combination was a huge hit for our Mr. Wonderful! Feeding him both tuna and chicken at once was a great food game.

July 8th: This was a very difficult day. Oscar was very sick with diarrhea, and was extremely weak from the illness. He was unable to eat anything all day long... We are on a roller coaster in helping him, and these low days are challenging in every way...That afternoon, Oscar climbed the back hill with me, and we just sat there in silence. (Winston stayed close to the house in the shade.) Although unable to eat, Oscar seemed so alert, and I was overwhelmed with sadness and frustration in not knowing what to do to help him. I felt so powerless and helpless, and in the peace and comfort of being alone with him and our beautiful trees, I started to cry. I let go, and allowed myself to sob out loud. I told Oscar that I wanted so very much to do more to help him. His eyes blinked, but his gaze never left my face. I reached over and hugged him close for the longest time. Then, we sat there quietly, taking in the beauty and majesty of the glorious beech tree. We sat there in silence for a long time...As the day moved along, Richard and I continued to do all that the day required. Then came the big surprise that brought a very happy ending to the day! At 9 p.m., Oscar came upstairs to get me after he heard the squeak from the armoire door opening where I keep my walking clothes. This had been his routine for the longest time, but to experience it on *this* day? With his tail wagging and his body squirming with delight I realized that he wanted to go for a walk! I just couldn't refuse him. Although not having eaten all day, Oscar did beautifully...We took our 16th three-mile walk that evening, and yes, they stopped to eat the special green leaves.

July 9th: Tonight, I offered Oscar a piece of shrimp at the end of our dinner. I thought it unlikely that he would want to eat it, but thought I would try. He licked his lips (oh, how he used to love shrimp), endured watching Winston devour his, and then walked past us to leave the room. I followed him and captured him with a huge hug...This was so heartbreaking. That evening, I had another dream. It began with Richard saying, "Look at Oscar! He's acting *confused*." I began to focus intently on Oscar, and monitored him constantly. He was rushed into a room closed off to me, and he clawed at the door to get out in a panic! I pulled him out of the room in the last second of time. The dream ended, and then there was peace.

July 10th: It is 60 days past the diagnosis, and Oscar is still alive! We live in the moment and celebrate with grateful hearts. Incredibly, tonight we took our 17th three-mile walk.

July 12th: This was a day filled with both love and anguish. We took our 18th three-mile walk. Eating the leaves has become a ritual for Oscar and Winston.

July 14th: I made a fresh batch of Oscar's newest food mixture. I combined three pounds of 80% lean, browned and drained Angus beef, with four slices of honey wheat bread, one loaf of Pepperidge Farm soft French bread, and four asiago bagels (all breads are cut-up)... Richard started a new tradition of bringing home a plain Chick-fil-A sandwich for Oscar's "lunch," and Oscar has happily adapted to the routine. When Oscar hears the garage door going up he dashes through the doggy door in the sunroom, and meets Richard in their secret hideout: by his food bowl in the third garage. (This way, Winston doesn't see or know about it. Then, again, maybe he does, but doesn't show it?) After eating, Oscar jumps back through the doggy door and returns to his favorite position in the family room. Right now, on his best days, Oscar is eating three meals.

July 15th: I discovered a fabulous new dog treat at the drug store today: carob sandwich cookies with a creamy vanilla filling. My goodness, these cookies are a phenomenal hit with Oscar!

July 18th: We weighed Oscar today, and he's up six pounds! He's back to weighing 82 pounds! In order to keep up with Oscar's appetite this week, I roasted another nine whole chickens. Richard and I agree that the leaves may have something to do with it. I want to learn everything I can about these leaves ASAP!

July 19th: One of the village tree consultants met with me today to identify the leaves and trees that have drawn Oscar's interest. He said it was some type of elm tree, but which kind? He wasn't certain due to the huge number of varieties. Much to my delight, he and I were able to identify two such elm trees in our front yard, including the majestic old tree with the glorious trunk along the road! The bark on these elm trees all looked different due to their varied ages... I wanted to experiment. Would Oscar want to eat the leaves from the trees in our front yard? I brought some leaves from the largest tree over to Oscar and to Winston, but they both appeared disinterested...It seems they only want the tender leaves from the seedlings found along our walking route, or those growing by the prominent roots of older, established trees...Tonight, Oscar begged for a 4th meal before heading upstairs at bedtime!... I stayed up quite late to research online about this particular elm tree. I hoped I might be able to identify its name by finding a photograph of a tree with the same glorious bark. My efforts were rewarded. Several Google searches resulted in the discovery of some fascinating information.

Amazingly, Oscar had discovered Slippery Elm leaves. Long recognized as an effective medicine and noted for its nutritional benefits, Slippery Elm is an FDA-approved, nonprescription soothing agent recommended for internal use.

The historical use of Slippery Elm goes all the way back to the days of the American Revolution. Rich in nutrients, surgeons used it to treat gunshot wounds. It was made into a broth or into gruel. In fact, George Washington and his troops survived on Slippery Elm gruel for several days during the harsh winter at Valley Forge when supplies could not reach them. Early American settlers also used it as a survival food (www.MDidea.com).

Native American Indian tribes are credited with discovering the healing substance within the inner bark of these majestic trees. Typically, it was pounded into a powder and then combined with water to create a multi-purpose healing substance. The powdered bark was given to people that could not keep any food down, and was also recommended for individuals losing weight and seemingly wasting away (www.MDidea.com).

In 1922, a Canadian nurse named Rene Caisse met an elderly woman who had been cured from cancer by an herbal tea remedy. Thirty years earlier, the woman had been diagnosed with breast cancer, but she was healed after following an herbal formula recommended by an old Native American Indian medicine man. The patient shared this herbal tea recipe with Nurse Caisse who refined the formula as she watched its effects on thousands of cancer patients over a 50-year career (www.healthfreedom.info). It was interesting to read that some of her patients gave the actual tea dregs (the herb particles that settle on the bottom of a jar of the herbal tea) to their pets or farm animals, and reported the same or similar results as humans had experienced!

One of the main ingredients of this herbal tea is the soft, inner white bark of the American Slippery Elm tree. Known as Essiac (Caisse spelled backwards) tea, there are many patient and doctor testaments recorded as public documents that attest to its effectiveness as a treatment for cancer (www.healthfreedom.info). Nurse Caisse protected her tea formula, and shared it with no one except the staff member who prepared the herbs for the tea administered at the cancer clinic. In 1994, prior to her death, this employee, who was also Renee's best friend, filed a handwritten affidavit that attested to the actual herbs and the proper methods to make the authentic Essiac tea.

Today, the United Plant Savers Association has found it necessary to place the American Slippery Elm tree on the endangered species list. Once thought to be resistant to the destructive Dutch elm disease that destroyed the vast number of American Elm trees, experts now know otherwise. The association recommends specific procedures for harvesting from the rare and resilient Slippery Elms that have survived, as protective measures must be taken. They advise harvesting only from the bark of the largest branches of the tree. Cutting bark from the main trunk "*may kill this stately tree that has given of itself so generously (www.MDidea.com).*"

Oscar had discovered just what he needed! The revelation was too remarkable for words. *All this time we have been searching for the meaning of this journey. Now we knew...*

July 20th: Oscar and Winston tiptoed downstairs to lay side by side in front of us tonight, while Richard and I were watching a movie. This was a first-ever happening as the routine has been for Winston to claim the area in front us, leaving Oscar to find a hiding place somewhere behind us. But here they were, lying still and peacefully...together.

Incredibly, earlier today we took our 20th three-mile walk, and there was a lot of leaf eating.

❧ The Catalog Arrives

July 21st: Oscar was unable to eat the chicken and rice mixture today. He was, however, able to eat plenty of plain roast chicken plus Milkbones cookies and some carob sandwich cookies. It wasn't that we wanted to give him cookies; we offered them only when he was disinterested in everything else. They were a last resort...Mary Rhodes suggested giving

Oscar some canned pumpkin to ease the nausea and diarrhea as it had worked so well for her dog. I appreciated the suggestion, and eagerly tried it, but, unfortunately, Oscar was disinterested. However, our sweet and adorable Winston was only too happy to eat it all up without a moment's pause.

July 22nd: Today was a poor-eating-day that became better. Oscar ate just a couple of small pieces of broiled chicken breast in the a.m., and only a piece or two of canned salmon at noon, so I went back to the current standby: roast chicken with no rice. He was quite eager to eat some roasted chicken. Wanting to keep up the calories, I decided to play a food game using small Milkbones cookies. Instead of handing them to him one at a time, I put the treats in his food bowl. Sure enough! He ate 20 flavored Milkbones…Later on, during our own dinner, Richard wondered if Oscar's appetite might be stimulated with something new and completely different. He suggested that we offer Oscar some roasted duck. (We had ordered a takeout Peking Duck dinner from a local Chinese restaurant that evening.) He called to Oscar, and Oscar came over to see what was going on at the dinner table. Richard offered him a piece of the duck, and he eagerly ate it, devouring all of the pieces remaining on Richard's plate. Because of this success, we decided to call-in a takeout order for Oscar at the Chinese restaurant. The employees found this to be quite amusing! Much to our delight, Oscar devoured the slices of freshly roasted duck mixed with just a little plum sauce. He even purred when he was finished. Later on in the evening, he ate 10 more small Milkbones… We took our 21st three-mile walk tonight and both dogs ate many of the Slippery Elm leaves which they now also have found in other locations along our walking route…Richard and I cherish all of these precious, simple moments of happiness.

    July 23rd: This day was a back-to-normal eating day for Oscar. The a.m. feeding included chicken with rice, and at noon he ate cut-up pieces of beef in its natural juices…In the afternoon, when I offered Winston a beef-basted rawhide strip, Oscar came over for one, too. This was new behavior—he had lost interest in rawhides when he became sick. I watched him as he climbed the hill in the backyard with Winston, lay down and then began licking the rawhide, eventually chewing on the ends. This was an improvement! He was now able to ingest the rawhide; he hadn't been able to do this since the diagnosis…In the p.m. feeding, he had a small portion of the chicken with rice.

    July 24th: This was a day of struggling. Oscar was incapable of eating much of anything. His eating has been up and down for four days now, and I'm very concerned that we have lost our grip on the battle for wellness. We continue to remind each other that this is one of the manifestations of cancer. This is an up and down journey. We can only cope by taking it one day at a time…We wish we could find a product that would treat his needs! We have such high expectations for ourselves…Oscar ate 12 small Milkbones (placed in his food bowl for the a.m. feeding), 1 ½ asiago bagels at noon and a plain Chick-fil-A sandwich for dinner.

    July 25th: Oscar and Winston had their bath and grooming appointments today. When we returned home, I brought in the mail, and discovered a new catalog. It was from a store by the name of the Only Natural Pet Store and it was located in Boulder, Colorado.

I held the catalog in my hands, knowing the timing of its arrival was by no means an accident. Anticipating that I would discover a product or remedy that would benefit Oscar, I opened it and began to read… and…One product that caught my attention was the Only Natural Pet GI Support and was described as being "ideal for animals suffering from chronic or recurrent poor digestion, food allergies, or irritable bowel issues, (catalog page 27)" and it contained *Slippery Elm bark*!

The product was made in an FDA-approved facility using human-grade ingredients, and was considered to be helpful in healing an impaired digestive system (the symptoms listed included vomiting and diarrhea). The 80+ ratings raved about its effectiveness! The product was composed of probiotics, vitamins, herbs, health-building co-factors and enzymes. This seemed to be an amazing remedy!

Another product, the Only Natural Pet Immune Strengthener, also merited consideration. Described as "a holistic combination of natural vitamins, minerals, herbs, and mushrooms to provide support to the immune system of dogs and cats fighting a chronic disease. Its synergistic ingredients include Vitamin C, Selenium, Coenzyme Q10, Astragalus, Cat's Claw, Green Tea Leaf, and much more. This powerful formula also includes Reishi, Shitake and Maitake mushrooms, three of the most commonly used mushrooms in Chinese herbal medicine (catalog page 29)."

Without hesitation, I picked up my phone and called the Only Natural Pet Store to place our first order.

July 26th: Thanks to the efficiency of overnight delivery, the Only Natural Pet GI Support and the Only Natural Pet Immune Strengthener arrived as expected this morning, and I began to administer the capsules to Oscar immediately. The instructions suggested sprinkling the contents of the capsules on top of the dog's food. I made a fresh batch of the drained, lean ground beef and bread mixture, and sprinkled the contents of the capsules on top of his food as the directions suggested, but it didn't work. Oscar refused to eat his food. So, I started over. I gave the capsules to him orally by placing them, one at a time, in the back of his mouth, and rewarded him with a treat after each. There was no resistance as this was how he'd always taken any meds. Besides, he seemed to understand that I was trying to help him. I gave him plenty of cuddles through it all…Both the a.m. and noon feedings went well, and he eagerly ate the warmed ground beef with bread mixture. However, he refused the mixture in the p.m. feeding so we quickly substituted leftover chicken with mashed potatoes. Later on, he ate 16 small Milkbones treats that we put in his food bowl.

July 28th: "Picky eating" continues, and we keep trying to offer foods until Oscar finds something that he can or wants to eat. We try to stimulate his palate through food games and creative maneuvers. The combination that worked today was a can of tuna in water over a cup of dry dog food with five flavored Milkbones cookies, arranged in a circle, on top. Oscar was very happy to play this newest food game…What also matters is that he seems happier! Sadly, though, we realize the weight gain from last week has again been lost. Nevertheless, we keep our hopes up! Following the recommendations and guidelines on each of the new products' labels, we continue to administer the appropriate dosages each day to Oscar…We took our 22nd three-mile walk, and *the Slippery Elm leaves continue to be the big attraction.*

July 29th: The day began slowly for Oscar, and he refused all food except for plain Milkbones treats. We are careful not to force food on him, but with kindness continue to try to offer him food. Could it be time for something new? Richard took charge. Surprise! Oscar ate 1 ½ plain, unsalted hamburger patties from Wendy's for lunch…The p.m. feeding was also a good report—we ordered a roasted duck from the Chinese restaurant, and he ate ¾ of the entire duck (cut into pieces) that was mixed with half an asiago bagel and ¼ cup of dry dog food.

It is essential for a dog caregiver to be able to respond to a sick dog's rejection of food with a thick-skinned mindset. One cannot interpret it as a personal rejection. Additionally, there is a delicate balance to managing the whole issue of eating: we didn't want to force him to eat, and yet we knew that if we didn't continue to offer various foods to Oscar, he wouldn't be able to survive. However, we also needed to recognize that there would be moments, and even, perhaps, an entire day (or days), when he would be unable to eat anything.

Everything about Oscar indicated that he wanted to live and overcome this disease. We tried very hard to match our efforts precisely to his mood and his ability to eat. In time, we were able to accept the eating versus non-eating, and kept right on loving him and praising him for other reasons. In the meantime, Winston kept a steadfast watch over everything, and continued to be a protective littermate when they were inside.

July 31st: We are thrilled! Oscar's been taking the supplements for five days, and they seem to be having a positive effect!! Oscar eagerly ate 2 asiago bagels with a full can of tuna in water for his a.m. feeding, skipped eating at noon, and his p.m. feeding was 1½ plain Chick-fil-A sandwiches served *Richard's-style*...Oscar continues to allow me to administer the supplements orally as previously described.

August 1st: Flavored Milkbones continue to be Oscar's choice for the morning feeding. We continue to entice him to eat, and he ate tuna with cut-up pieces of asiago bagels today. He manages to take the capsules easily throughout the day and happily accepts a treat after each one is swallowed.

August 2: We took our 23rd three-mile walk around 9:30 p.m., but Winston blocked Oscar from taking the shortcut home. Was this change on Oscar's part due to the heat? I wonder.

August 3rd-5th: I'm away visiting relatives, and attending a conference in Florida. Richard assumed the responsibility for caring for Oscar and Winston, and all went along well, *Richard's-style*.

August 6th: This was a poor eating day. I offered Oscar broiled chicken, roasted chicken, and his favorite cookies, but all offerings yielded no response. Finally, lamb drew his interest. It is becoming increasingly difficult (humanly impossible) to have enough alternatives of home-cooked food on hand to manage Oscar's needs. Richard brought home plain, unsalted hamburgers and some takeout lamb. Oscar ate it all!

August 7th: Eating went more easily today. I made some French toast using good Italian bread for his morning feeding, and he ate it eagerly. At noon he ate pieces of chicken breast. His p.m. feeding was a Wendy's hamburger served *Richard's-style*.

August 8th: Amazingly, we took our 25th three-mile walk today. All went OK.

I am so grateful for Richard's unique and most excellent way of helping in Oscar's healing journey. It brings me great joy to watch them during their precious feeding moments.

↬ Wingalings, Smothered Comfort and Working Dog's Stew

August 9th: Eating problem intensifies: Oscar is refusing to eat any more home-prepared foods. I searched through several stores for high protein treats and keep these on hand for emergencies, and also to reward him after each of his supplements. This morning, I put flavored Milkbones in his bowl with his vitamin, and he ate 11 treats for his a.m. feeding. Another new treat, Nutsters, has become appealing to him (peanut butter flavor) and he ate ½ of the jar for his p.m. feeding. Richard and I are unsure about what to try next. I bought the food our vet recommended, but it, too, was refused... Oscar ate many of the new soft chicken-flavored Milkbones treats upstairs prior to going to sleep.

As I went through my e-mails that evening, I noticed one from the

Only Natural Pet Store regarding a relevant product for dog cancer by the name of PhytoPharmica Cellular Forte with IP-6 & Inositol. The description of item 106001 read, " A dietary supplement to enhance natural killer-cell activity and boost the immune system. Cellular Forte is the only patented combination of IP-6 and Inositol." I decided to order 120 capsules of this product.

I also decided to order some cases of very charming all-natural canned dog food. The names of the varieties alone sounded creative and delicious—the perfect mix for Oscar's palate! Wingalings, Smothered Comfort, and Working Dog Stew? How about Dog Food Lunch Box, Turducken, Mediterranean Banquet, and Harvest Moon? The names of the Merrick canned dog food were delightful, and I hope Oscar (and Winston) will agree!! I placed a rather large order. Due to its weight, the cost of overnight shipping would have been more than an airline ticket – we'll need to be patient for our order to arrive via Standard UPS delivery. In the meantime, whatever Oscar wants to eat is better than eating nothing.

August 10th: Today, it is three months since Oscar's diagnosis. He was quite lethargic today. I wondered if he might be experiencing any pain, and decided to give him a Rimadyl to see if he responded accordingly. According to Dr. Heller, there was no indication that Oscar was in any pain, and he certainly didn't seem to appear to feel any better after taking the Rimadyl. Flavored Milkbones and Nutsters in his dog food bowl were what appealed to him today, that is, until Richard came home with a plain Chick-fil-A sandwich. Even then, he ate the chicken without the bread. However, his spirits picked up after that, and he came over to nudge me with his cold nose later while we were watching a movie. I took Oscar and Winston outside to walk around the backyard. I gazed up into the starry night and focused on the day. I prayed for continued strength and wisdom for the journey and trusted that the new Merrick dog food would arrive at the best possible moment.

August 11th: This was an absolutely great day! The morning feeding consisted of Nutsters in his bowl, and he ate them eagerly. The product label indicates that it has good protein content. Oscar was his usual self—abounding with happiness, shredding the Kleenex from the bathroom trash can, and walking around with his baby gorilla toy in his mouth. At noon, I put more Nutsters into his bowl, and he enticed Winston into a competition before eating them. His evening feeding included some cut-up lamb with four flavored Milkbones. After he had his four capsules, he ate 25-30 more Nutsters.

August 12th: Today, Oscar ate lamb at noon. At his p.m. feeding he gobbled three mouthfuls of lamb, walked away and then vomited it all up. Today, it seemed that he ate just to please us. At 9 p.m., Richard went out to pick-up a plain grilled chicken sandwich which he offered to Oscar, *Richard's style*...We took our 26th three-mile walk, and *both dogs eagerly pulled me down the hill in anticipation of the patch of Slippery Elm leaves!*

August 13th: We're struggling, but at least Oscar's eating something. At 9:30 am Oscar ate Nutsters plus his supplements and four flavored Milkbones. His noon feeding consisted of a plain Chick-fil-A without the bun, and he ate two plain Chick-fil-A's for dinner served *Richard's-*

style without the soft bun. The good news is that he continues to take his supplements without any resistance, and he seems quite content to receive a flavored Milkbone after each.

August 14th: I called Dr. Heller's office today to renew Winston's Rimadyl prescription and again, they were amazed to hear about Oscar. Joyce Carrick encouraged me to write a story about this to help other dog owners, and I truly believe that one day I will. Joyce said, "Oscar knew what he needed." I do so appreciate her support and encouragement! Eating today continued in the same pattern as the past few days: 12 flavored Milkbones at 8 a.m., ⅔ bowl of Nutsters at noon plus all of his supplements, and nearly 2 ½ Chick-fil-A sandwiches without the soft bun. At 9 p.m., Oscar and Winston wanted to take their walk, but due to Oscar's irregular eating I limited it to 1½ miles. But, of course, they ate the leaves!

August 15th: Today, brought a special moment for Richard! Oscar cuddled under his arm during breakfast and competed with Winston for pieces of the asiago bagel. We haven't seen this kind of interaction for the longest time…And, thanks to Winston's strong desire for the Nutsters he found in Oscar's food bowl, Oscar developed a sudden interest in eating. Before we knew it, all of the Nutsters were eaten!

August 16th: Hurray!!! Hurray!!! The boxes of Merrick canned dog food from the Only Natural Pet Store arrived just before dinner. They are a huge success! Oscar devoured 1½ cans of Wingaling (slow-cooked chicken wings) in addition to his supplements. He ate all that was in his bowl, and then licked the bowl *completely* clean (and Winston likewise).

It feels so good to have him eating healthy food again. These products were heaven sent… We ended the day with our three-mile walk.

August 17th-22nd: The new dog food has provided the backbone to Oscar's newest eating program; however, we continue to offer canned tuna with water with asiago bagels when Oscar is recovering from a bout of vomiting or diarrhea. He has found a new favorite spot to lie during the day: on the cool brick floor between the sunroom and the family room as the trickle of water from the sunroom fountain soothes him. Our weather has been very hot this week. As a result, we have had nightly thunderstorms that both dogs have always found to be high-stress experiences.

August 23rd and 24th: Discovered another new treat for Oscar today. They're called King Louis cookies, and they're made with peanut butter…Hot temperatures and thunderstorms continue, and we're up with Oscar every night now.

August 25th: What a good day this was! There were many happy moments. Winston lay down beside Oscar today and licked both of his ears clean—even their tails were wagging with joy! We haven't seen this interaction since before Oscar became ill.

There was another wonderful part to this day. Somewhere around 5:30-6 p.m., I noticed that Oscar was standing in front of a small, fenced in area between the house and garage in the backyard. He appeared to be eyeing something through a crack in the gate, and kept looking at me as if he wanted to go in there. I was interested in seeing what had captured his attention. As I opened the gate, Oscar and Winston went in and, a second or two later, Winston came out munching on some Slippery Elm leaves. (The evidence was all over his face!) Oscar was sniffing everywhere in earnest, and then, with much gusto, began to eat the Slippery Elm leaves from this new patch of seedlings he had discovered. He was having so much fun!

This was a very significant discovery as *this meant he could eat the leaves each day from the backyard*. I was filled with an unspeakable joy. What were the chances of having a tree from the endangered species list in one's front *and* back yard? I stood there watching them eating the leaves, and absorbed the significance of the moment.

This is Oscar's journey, and he is leading us. We are his students, and he is the teacher. I knelt down beside them and hugged them close; they soon found the tears streaming down my face and licked furiously to wipe them away. I wanted to hold onto the Light of the moment, but their silliness took over as they tumbled me over. *Yes, this is a difficult time for us, but the measure of love and joy far exceeds anything we could ever have imagined.*

August 28th: Our second shipment of the adorable Merrick canned dog food has arrived!

August 29th: Wingaling is clearly the favorite food of the week. Because of Merrick's slow-cooked method of preparation, the chicken bones, which are a natural source of calcium, may be eaten. It's obvious the dogs find this to be great fun! The Only Natural Pet Store catalog has been a treasure chest...True to his nature, Oscar is continuing to accept the new supplements. He knows that they are helping him. How do I know this? Tonight, while I was giving him his pills downstairs, I realized that I needed more treats to match the last two cell renewal tablets. I put the two tablets down on the carpet and ran upstairs into the kitchen to get more of his favorite cookies. When I returned, *I saw that he had eaten the last two tablets on his own. He was watching to see my reaction. Oh, beloved Oscar! You are forever full of surprises.*

With the addition of the canned dog food, additional supplements and new cookies we were able to maneuver the course more ably during the coming week. The dogs' bath and grooming appointments went along OK; the commotion from the heating and cooling workmen in and out for two days was difficult, but we remained flexible and chose to *flow with the moment, confident now that what Oscar needed would be provided.* Oscar continues to lose weight, but we are focusing on the positive aspects of the journey. Our job is to be connected to him at every step, and this brings everyone joy.

September 8th: Recently, our late night walks (despite Oscar's very thin physique, he still begs for a walk) have provided Oscar and Winston with additional stimulation and intrigue. The occasional viewing of a family of deer has become more frequent, and I find it quite interesting that Oscar and Winston stop walking when they notice the deer. They do so more in reverence than fear; the deer, in turn, do not flee the minute they notice the dogs.

Tonight, we had a double dose of excitement. First, there was the spotting of the doe and her two young deer. Oscar and Winston stopped suddenly and we stood quietly, dead center on a village road, listening to the sound of their hooves as they crossed a short distance in front of us. I reflected on this precious moment much too long this evening for, as we continued on, unbeknownst to me, another furry creature was approaching us on the other side of the street. The dogs must have sensed my preoccupied thoughts. To my great amazement, they both simultaneously crossed over to the other side of the road, leading the way, to avoid a face-to-face confrontation with a *skunk!!*

When I realized why they had moved to the other side of the road, I marveled at their wisdom and ability to navigate us away from a potential problem. In the past, they had treated skunks as if they were their stuffed squeaky toys, which resulted in many late night baths from being sprayed by the frightened and angered creatures. But, amazingly, this did not happen tonight!

My gratitude and love abounds, and I feel renewed for the next season.

CHAPTER TWO

Last Fall With Oscar

⁃ Cheering Him On!

With school in session for more than a week now, the feeling of fall was clearly in the air. The four young McKenna boys next door are great Oscar (and Winston) fans, and they continue to check on both dogs despite their evening homework and additional after-school activities. The neighbors in our small village have become accustomed to Oscar stopping and grazing as we walked during the summer months. Richard and I are profoundly grateful for their kindness and neighborly understanding as our dogs sniffed along the road on their properties hoping to find some more fresh Slippery Elm seedlings.

Word of Oscar's story had spread so far that cars would stop to say hi, and to check on him. Other walkers did the same. Oscar and Winston were accustomed to the interruptions, and fully enjoyed the attention. The Village police had come to know us as well through all of our walks. "Go, Oscar!" became the mantra from a female officer who patrolled on some weekends. Those officers who worked on the evenings we took our walks also stopped to cheer him on.

Oscar appeared very thin, but the strength of his conviction and determination to live resounded quite clearly.

September 9th: Oscar no longer wants to eat the sauce from the new canned dog food, and I suspect it may be aggravating his diarrhea. I tried pouring the canned food over rice, but he was disinterested. Remaining flexible, I switched to his love of bread for a solution. At noon he ate one can of tuna in water with pieces of soft rolls (slightly sweet) plus two slices of Italian bread cut into pieces. He gobbled it up! At 5 p.m., he ate a can of Wingaling poured over one large slice of cut-up Italian bread.

September 10th: Oscar ate poorly all day except for gobbling down bread and King Louis cookies. This was very hard to bear—at noon his raging hunger was obvious with loud growling noises from his stomach, and he was listless. We continued on with all of his supplements.

September 11th: This was a wonderful eating day! In the a.m. feeding, he had four slices of Sara Jane's honey wheat bread including his supplements. At noon, he ate one slice of Sara Jane's honey wheat bread on top of a can of Wingaling. I noticed that his stool was firmer today. At 4 p.m., we took our three-mile walk so that he could eat some Slippery Elm leaves. Upon our return home he ate almost two slices of honey wheat bread over a can of Wingaling plus his supplements. Later on, he ate slices of leftover roast chicken from our dinner, his capsules plus three large Milkbones and three King Louis cookies.

September 12th: The a.m. and noon feedings consisted only of honey wheat or Italian bread. I decided to call the Only Natural Pet

Store to see about any other suggestions, and they told me about the Only Natural Pet B.S.S.T. Herbal Formula that contains the four herbs in the well known Essiac tea formula: burdock root, sheep sorrel, Slippery Elm and turkey rhubarb root. According to their catalogue, "these herbs may help reduce tumor growth, purify blood, and carry away destroyed tissue. The formula helps strengthen the innate defense mechanisms of the body, enabling normal cells to destroy abnormal cells (catalog page 29)." I ordered two bottles along with refills of the other products we were using…I stopped by the Animal Care Clinic to pick-up some products for Winston, and again Joyce Carrick inquired about Oscar. I brought a list of all the products and remedies we were using to share with Dr. Heller; she was overjoyed, and indicated that this information would be so helpful to others dealing with dog cancer. "You must write a book about this," she stated firmly…Oscar's evening feeding was identical to yesterday with the addition of some large pieces of pork roast. He ate tonight as if he were well!

September 13th: In the a.m., Oscar ate two pieces of Sara Jane's honey wheat bread; at noon, he enjoyed one can of Wingaling plus one slice of honey-wheat bread and one soft dinner roll (the flavor is on the sweet side). As usual, supplements were worked into the day. The p.m. feeding was one can of Wingaling plus another piece of honey wheat bread followed by many cookies.

September 14th: In the a.m., Oscar ate two pieces of honey wheat bread plus chunks of leftover pork roast. At noon, he was eager to eat a can of Wingaling with one slice of honey wheat bread and one soft dinner roll followed by two small Milkbones and approximately eight

Nutsters. I am smiling as I write that "he wolfed down" one can of Wingaling with 1½ slices of honey wheat bread.

September 15th: In the morning, Oscar ate 3½ slices of honey wheat bread. At 2:30 p.m. and at 4:30 p.m., he ate a full can of Wingaling plus a slice of honey wheat bread and one soft dinner roll. Oscar and Winston begged for a walk so we ventured out to do our favorite three-mile trek through the Village. We had fun making a game of eating the Slippery Elm leaves today! I stopped, bent down to pretend that I was interested in the leaves, and Oscar immediately grabbed the largest Slippery Elm leaves he could reach. He ate five or six large leaves very quickly before eating others at a grazing pace. Meanwhile, Winston ate the leaves voraciously while Oscar and I played, and this concerns me.

September 17th: We are so encouraged with the increased stability in Oscar's eating pattern. The combination of foods and most of the remedies appear to be effective. Unfortunately, we are uncertain about the B.S.S.T. product's use for Oscar. Drops are to be added to the dog's water (i.e., several drops into the water bowl), but Oscar detected a difference in his water and stopped drinking the water from the bowl… In the morning, he ate 4½ slices of honey wheat bread on top of ⅓ c. of dry dog food. At noon, he was only too happy to eat a can of Smothered Comfort (slow-cooked chicken thighs with delightful extras) plus one slice of honey wheat bread. Finally, his evening meal consisted of two cans of Smothered Comfort with only a tablespoon or two of the gravy (it may cause him to have a loose stool) plus 1½ slices of Sara Jane's honey wheat bread (available at our local health food store)…Tonight, I received an extra dose of licks after Oscar's prayer. We offer him as many cookies as he wants to eat. How can a dog sleep well if his stomach is growling with hunger?

September 18-19th: The 18th was another great eating day. However, the next day, Oscar began his day with two-plus pieces of honey wheat bread with four chunks of chicken breast and then surprised us by vomiting up bile. We comforted him throughout the remainder of the day.

September 20th: Oscar only wanted to eat the small flavored Milkbones this morning but happily ate between 12-15 treats. Richard brought him a plain Wendy's hamburger at noon (done *Richard's-style and in their secret place*), and in the evening I was overjoyed to note that he ate three cans of Wingalings without the gravy but with the extra carrots, etc., plus his supplements and some bread. Later, he had two slices of Italian bread plus two more capsules...Oscar and Winston wanted to go for a walk, and of course, I consented. However, I cut it short at one and a third miles.

September 21st: Oscar was able to eat one slice of honey wheat bread plus one soft dinner roll. Interestingly, I was able to hand feed him two honey wheat rolls that were dipped in Smothered Comfort Sauce. He then ate the chicken thigh with the supplements sprinkled on top. This is the first time he was willing to take his supplements this way!

September 22nd: This was an especially good day despite the intense heat. Oscar's morning meal was comprised of one and a half slices of honey wheat bread. At 11 a.m., I fed him most of the can of Wingaling, a honey wheat roll and his supplements, and at 6 p.m., he ate a full can of Smothered Comfort with one and a half honey wheat rolls dipped in the gravy with his supplements. This new way of administering his supplements (rewarding him with a piece of the roll dipped in the gravy) is providing him with extra nutrition. Later on in the evening, he ate some leftovers from our evening meal: pieces of veal, some kugel (baked egg noodles) and some King Louis cookies after each of his capsules.

September 23rd: Oscar's morning vitamin and cookies have become a daily constant. I believe this is as comforting to Winston as it is to Oscar. Oscar didn't seem to want any bread today (?). His morning meal consisted of 13 flavored Milkbones. At noon, I fed him two pieces of veal, two King Louis peanut butter cookies and one large Milkbone. At 8 p.m., he ate a full can of Wingaling plus his supplements. He sprang through the doggy door to head outside with a large Milkbone in his mouth!

September 24th: Oscar woke me this morning with a "whole" spirit of energy, and I drew in the beauty and joy of the moment. He radiates love and Light!

September 25th: Oscar ate 14 flavored Milkbones for his morning meal, and ate honey wheat bread and supplements at noon. The dogs had their bath and grooming appointments this afternoon. Oscar and Winston love getting in the car to go places, so this is a good thing! In the evening, Oscar ate two cans of Smothered Comfort without the gravy.

September 26th: I read about the NF Spectra Probiotic product on the Only Natural Pet Store's website (www.onlynaturalpet.com) today. The description noted, "NF's Spectra Probiotic is a well-tolerated multi-probiotic formula that provides both beneficial intestinal bacteria and growth factors known to promote recolonization…" Among its listed areas of effectiveness are two areas applicable to Oscar's condition: aids in digestion and suppressing disease-causing bacteria, and aids in preventing and treating diarrhea. I decided to order 90 capsules of the product.

As I wrote this entry, I realized we didn't have a data entry in the log for September 26th and 27th, and this merits an explanation. My work as a forensic behavioral scientist has blended me into the world of intelligence and homeland security, and I was preparing to take the Level lV Course & Examination along with the Level V Course & Examination (the highest attainment) at the American Board for Certification in Homeland Security National Conference the first week of October. Additionally, I was the invited banquet keynote speaker, which meant that I was writing, researching and studying at all hours of the day. I was living through one of the most demanding times of my professional life—I remember how hard it was for Richard to manage my schedule—surely, my personal stress was affecting Oscar and Winston.

This was my first keynote speech, and I put my heart and soul into writing it. Entitled, "Aspiring to the Best Practices Standard," the speech was an invitation for the audience to join me in exploring the possibility of bringing change to the world by very simply expecting more from others and expecting more from ourselves, my definition of the best practices standard of living. The perspective I wanted to share was a discovery that has resulted from much overcoming, and a life that has been, by circumstance and by choice, an uphill climb.

The underpinning of this perspective is supported by significant research findings on the positive and negative effects of expectations. Rich data suggests that the power of expectations is subtly at work all the time. Expectations of self and others have much to do with achievement, overcoming adversity and successfully navigating life's challenges. "Aspiring to a Best Practice Standard *of Living*," then, presents unlimited possibilities! This new outlook activates a power that is amazingly exciting. What might happen if individually and collectively we were to channel this power? Indeed, a new level of expectations for ourselves, for those we love and with whom we work brings a fresh new field of energy, a new momentum, and a new set of lenses from which to grow, share life, create solutions and rebuild our world! I felt better after working on my speech tonight.

During a quiet moment of reflection, I realized that writing and believing in my own speech brought me the reassurance I needed: If I expect I can do it, I will be able to do so. Indeed, I was capable of completing everything well even as I also cared for Oscar. Keep going!

✒ Managing the Strain

One manages strain more easily and has an increased capacity to endure by believing that God is always there for us, and His supernatural powers are always working to help us. We are not alone with our burden. There was never a moment that Richard and I didn't believe God had brought this journey into our lives for a very good reason, even on days when there wasn't enough time, sleep, the right food "match" for Oscar, or energy to go around. Little breaks came here or there, plus we received cheerful support from those who cared about us. Most people seemed to relate to our bond of love with our beloved Oscar.

However, there were some who didn't understand why we chose not to euhanize Oscar when there really was no concrete possibility that he would ever recover. They couldn't see the value of time well spent in what we were doing. These people would make poking comments and would frown with concern and disapproval when we would be in their proximity. They did not share the same regard for how people and animals should be treated. When our paths crossed with such-minded individuals, I realized that our choice to help Oscar live was a reminder of another way to manage dog cancer. Oscar's very thin physique was painful to observe, but he was still living a high quality of life. Euthanizing him was out of the question.

Additional strain resulted from not knowing if Oscar was going to be here another day, week, month, or whether he might die later that evening. Anticipatory loss and anticipatory anxiety traveled on the journey with us. When my work took me away from home, I suffered privately with concern that he might die before I was able to return home.

To all situations, perspectives and scenarios there was always one source of comfort that enabled a greater ability to manage the strain. That was faith:

God knows all and is in charge of all. What I needed to do was to focus on loving. And that was easy for me to do.

September 28th: The pattern today clearly shows that Oscar's eating habits are again weakening.

September 29th: Oscar ate 16 flavored Milkbones plus one slice of Pane Turano (Italian) bread plus his supplements. He ate nothing at noon. We went for a walk at 4:30 p.m. By 6:30 p.m., he appeared to be hungry, and ate his dinner of Pane Turano bread with one can of Smothered Comfort dog food. We continue to administer all of the supplements from the four products and believe them to be extremely effective.

September 30th: In the morning, Oscar ate 16 flavored Milkbones, along with his supplements, as well as a slice of Pane Turano (Italian) bread, and at noon he ate the pieces of one honey wheat roll. In the evening, he ate two cans of Wingaling with one slice of Pane Turano, flavored Milkbones and his supplements...Today, I wrote out detailed instructions about feeding and supplement times, labeled the products and made certain that enough varieties of food and cookies for Oscar and Winston were in the house. Richard jokingly commented to friends that Oscar's feeding and medication schedules are as complicated as a human's... I am so grateful for his commitment to keep on loving Oscar until the end. I privately acknowledged my reluctance to leave for the entire week, but we both realize this is what I must do.

October 1st: Richard began full-time care for the dogs today as I am away in Kansas City, Kansas for a full week of work. Thankfully, he remembered to take notes each day. Today, Oscar ate 15 flavored Milkbone cookies, Pane Turano bread plus four of his supplements in the morning. At lunch, he ate a soft dinner roll... Unfortunately, the shrill alarm system went off today due to the weather conditions. The poor dogs! In the evening, Oscar ate two full cans of Wingaling with pieces of Pane Turano bread...Richard also gave into their wagging-tails' request for a night-time walk! There was a lot of leaf eating.

October 2nd: In the morning, Oscar ate 13 cookies and three supplements with honey wheat bread. At noon, he ate one dinner roll plus cookies, and the evening consisted of a full can of Wingaling with Pane Turano bread plus his supplements.

October 3rd: This was an unusual a.m. feeding: Oscar wanted a piece of Richard's apple pastry (of course, Winston got a piece, too), one supplement with honey wheat bread, 15 cookies and four supplements. At noon, Oscar only ate two pieces of bread, but for dinner he ate a can of Wingaling plus his supplements. Later, he ate a piece of Pane Turano bread with the cellular forte, and had fun eating two King Louis cookies.

October 4th: Oscar ate two whole pieces of honey wheat bread plus his supplements for the a.m. feeding, two soft dinner rolls at noon, and at dinner two full cans of Wingaling with two pieces of Pane Turano bread. Richard also took them on an evening walk. Before heading up to bed, Oscar ate two honey wheat rolls, one King Louis cookie and his cellular forte tablet.

October 5th: In the morning, Oscar (and Winston) ate a piece of Richard's blueberry muffin, his supplements, part of an asiago bagel and a few cookies. At noon, he had 1½ asiago bagels, and at dinner he ate a can of Wingaling with two pieces of Pane Turano bread plus *some pizza crust*. Later on, Oscar ate more pizza crust plus some King Louis cookies with his cellular forte tablet.

October 6th: In the morning, Oscar ate 12 cookies plus one piece of Pane Turano bread along with his supplements. At noon, he ate a Chick-fil-A in his hideout *Richard's-style*. His p.m. feeding consisted of two cans of Smothered Comfort with Pane Turano bread plus supplements.

October 7th: The a.m. feeding was a simple five flavored Milkbones cookies with his supplements plus one large slice of Pane Turano bread. In the afternoon he ate two slices of honey wheat bread with one can of Wingaling.

October 9th: There was much chaos around the house today due to the installation of our new generator...The NF Spectra Probiotic is working, but my big concern is now on Oscar's mood change. The strain of fighting the disease is fatiguing and emotionally draining. How can we help lift some of the burden from him? I reassured him with love all day long. He has always responded to hugs and has needed more than most dogs. Thankfully, the day ended more brightly for Oscar. Winston remained close to him all day long.

October 10th: I saw Oscar eating small bits of mud at the top of the hill today, and I wondered if he missed the texture of the dry dog food.

The sauces from of gourmet dog food may be aggravating his diarrhea right now. He was disinterested in cookies today, so I gave him 1½ cups of dry dog food with 2½ pieces of Pane Turano bread *and he ate it all. His evening meal consisted of 3+ cups of dry dogfood!* This is so encouraging.

October 11th: Oscar ate two cups of dry dog food in the morning, 1½ slices of Pane Turano bread at noon, and two cans of Wingaling with two slices of honey wheat bread for his evening feeding.

October 12th: It is cool and rainy today. Unfortunately, Oscar didn't eat anything during the morning or at noon except for a couple of small Milkbones treats and the NF Spectra Probiotic. He wanted to rest in the dog bed area of our third garage, and I nestled-him-in cozily and covered him with soft towels…Surprise! For dinner he ate two cans of Wingaling with 1½ honey-wheat dinner rolls.

October 17th: The past few days have been busy with the end of fall yard tasks. Before the workmen arrived this morning to bring in the large plants and trees that had been on the patio this summer, *Oscar ate three cups of dry dog food with his supplements. At 5 p.m., he ate two cans of Wingaling plus pieces of Pane Turano bread. Then, at 8 p.m. he ate an additional 2½ cups dry dog food plus two cans of Wingaling!*

October 20th: I love the memory of this moment. When I left today, I noticed that Oscar was out in the backyard watching me back my car out of the garage. Just like old times! He would always jump through the doggy door (for some reason, Winston always needed someone to hold the door open before he would jump through) to watch me leave.

He would watch for my car to return home, and when he saw my car in the driveway he would jump back into the sunroom just as he heard the garage door going up…His evening meal reflected an increased capacity to eat: I didn't need to dip the bread or roll into the sauce to entice him. I also hid the supplements, and sprinkled some under the chicken wings and other Wingaling ingredients. Today, he seems much stronger!

October 21st: This was a very difficult day. Oscar greatly suffered all day with diarrhea.

October 22nd: It was hard for Oscar to spring back today. Additionally, he is sensitive to noise, and workmen began working next door today on an addition to our neighbor's home. Oscar's eating patterns have returned to the pattern of earlier months; it's a struggle getting him to eat, but he waits for me to encourage him to try to eat.

October 23rd: It rained all day long today. The season is progressing, and the rain is pounding away on the remaining Slippery Elm leaves. I am growing quite concerned about the dogs' response to not being able to eat any more leaves (when they fall off of the seedlings).

October 24th: Richard will be gone for most of the week, and I decide to introduce Oscar to a new food at dinner. For his morning feeding he ate pieces of toast and his supplements, and the same occurred at noon. For his p.m. feeding, I offered Oscar (and Winston) something new: rotisserie chicken, and it was an enormous hit! Oscar ate nearly the entire chicken without any bread, rolls or dry dog food…I left both the sunroom lights and the outdoor lights on for Oscar tonight so that he could come and go as he needs to (during stretches of diarrhea, he seems to want to sleep on the cool family room floor as well).

October 25th: This morning Oscar was unable to eat anything. Around 2 p.m., he ate some leftover rotisserie chicken with a piece of bread…To help relieve his boredom, we created another new game. I gave Winston a large beef-basted rawhide, but as Oscar couldn't have one he received a huge piece of Pane Turano bread instead. For a moment, both dogs stared at each other, and then Oscar began to act silly by parading around with it in his mouth. Believe me, Winston kept watch as he licked his rawhide quite furiously. Rest assured, I made sure they both were OK as they enjoyed separate-but-equal treats…Finally, at dinner, Oscar ate well again! He ate two full cans of Smothered Comfort dog food with his supplements along with ½ cup of dry dog food plus one slice of Pane Turano bread.

October 27th: This was a morning of many failed attempts to try to find something that Oscar would eat, but I finally succeeded when I offered him some ham. He then went on to eat 1½ slices of cut-up ham with two cups of dry dog food, and then at 4:50 p.m. he ate two full slices of cut-up ham with a half cup of dry dog food.

October 29th: *Winston* is very ill today and is vomiting and has diarrhea!… I reordered more food and supplies from the Only Natural Pet Store today. In the evening Oscar ate his complete dinner plus two large Milkbones…We have great concerns about Winston, but as he has always been adventurous regarding what he has eaten, we are holding back on being alarmed that this could be serious. We'll keep a close watch on it.

October 30th: In the morning today, Oscar ate ½ of a slice of ham. Around noon, he ate the remainder of the slice of ham with 1½ slices of honey wheat bread. His evening feeding was excellent: 2 ½ cans of Wingaling with the sauce, and two full slices of Pane Turano bread... Thankfully, Winston seems to be doing better today.

October 31st: Happy Halloween! The day began with Oscar eating a dozen assorted small Milkbone cookies in his bowl. It is very cool and also a rainy day so Oscar spent his day indoors resting with Winston. I brought home two flavors of rotisserie chicken from another health food store, and Oscar devoured (Winston received a sample of each) both chickens during the remainder of the day...Interestingly, I found some empty wrappers of the small-size Pay Day candy bars in the foyer at the end of the day, and all indicators point to our precious Mr. Winston as the culprit. How he snuck those out of the basket of treats for the trick-or-treaters is amazing to me! That's our mischievous Mr. Winston!

November 3rd: The past few days have been consistent, excellent eating days for Oscar! This morning was exemplary: at 8:15 a.m., Oscar ate 2½ cups of dry dog food and his supplements, plus at least 1½ asiago rolls. His supplements are continuing to be effective—the weather has been cold and rainy, so we haven't taken walks for a while.

November 4th: In the a.m., Oscar ate one cup of dry dog food, and one cut-up ham slice at noon. Around 2:30 p.m., he begged for some pieces of the pepperoni bread others were eating, so he was given a couple of pieces in his bowl. Amazingly, he ate it all. This evening he ate two cans of Smothered Comfort with three medium-large slices of Pane Turano bread...Now for the surprise! He wanted his bowl filled *four* more times!!!!

November 5th: Things continue to move in a positive direction with Oscar's eating, but he is choosing to sleep alone downstairs in the family room. We leave the sunroom door open for him and leave the backyard lights on in the event he needs to go outside...Both dogs had their bath and grooming appointments today.

November 9th: The strong and healthy eating pattern continues for Oscar. This is the third night he ate three full cans of Wingaling at his evening feeding!!! We took our three-mile walk this evening, and both dogs stopped to eat the Slippery Elm leaves. I am so grateful they were still able to find some to eat!...Oscar continues to sleep downstairs.

The time grows close to when all the leaves will be gone. Will Oscar and Winston be able to manage their disappointment?

❧ The Leaves Fall Off

November 11th: Our precious Oscar continues to eat his vitamin in the morning, as does his doting littermate. This has been the routine since they were puppies! Oscar may not always eat his second small Milkbones cookie, *but he always eats his vitamin.* The evening prayer time is something they love. Oscar's deep sighs and fervent licks provide me with all the feedback I need to know this activity is comforting to him.

November 16-17th: These were very poor eating days! I am contemplating doing a food switch back to rice, again. In the p.m., Oscar ate three cans of Wingaling with 2¾ slices of honey wheat bread.

November 18th: In the morning, I offered Oscar one can of Wingaling with one cup of brown rice plus his supplements. Hurray! It worked! I was so relieved when he was interested in eating the new mixture. I understand that he is not rejecting me, but when he refuses to eat, it is a challenge to keep coming up with new food combinations. At noon, Oscar again ate one can of Wingaling with one cup of brown rice…The seasons are changing, and the weather has become our typical early winter Ohio weather. Most of the Slippery Elm leaves have fallen off, and both dogs grabbed at the last of them that were clinging to the seedlings. They both sniffed all over the empty branches (sniffing for the scent of fresh buds?) and seemed very anxious about not finding anymore anywhere! This was a sad moment for me to observe, but I told them encouragingly, "The leaves will be back! They'll come back in the spring."

But, would Oscar still be with us in the spring? It occurred to me that this was, perhaps, their last walk together when they would share in the eating of Slippery Elm leaves.

November 19th: Today, it was Winston's turn to have an appointment with Dr. Heller. The appointment was set up as his yearly examination, but as we'd noticed the intensity of his Slippery Elm leaf eating and other irregularities, we wanted to bring these concerns to Dr. Heller's attention. Fortunately, Winston was a true sport about the intensity of the probing, physical examination. But then, Dr. Heller's face turned grim. He found a 4"x12" mass that stretched from his stomach to his side. Are we going to lose them both? I mentioned to Dr. Heller that their father had died from a tumor when he was 8, but I didn't have any more facts. The test results will be available in a couple of days. We feel crushed with anticipatory sorrow, but press on and hold tight.

November 21st: Today is the day before Thanksgiving. Oscar had his own scheduled appointment with Dr. Heller, and Richard and Winston came with us as well. We sat there in the small examination room, all four of us, not knowing what news the next moment might bring. Dr. Heller entered the room and his kind, caring eyes reflected major concern and dismay. His first words to us were, "We still don't have the test results for Winston's tumor." Richard and I were slightly relieved to hear this, even though it just prolonged our not knowing. Never mind, there was more to attend to! Dr. Heller's attention turned toward Oscar, who, although his ribs were clearly showing, was sharing his love and Light. All the while Dr. Heller stated all of the grim medical details about Oscar's health, Oscar kept trying to leap-up to lick him and to share his joy... Dr. Heller emphasized that Oscar was anemic, and that his passing was near. He gave us a two-week dose of an appetite stimulant that he referred to as "dog hospice." Dog hospice begins today. The end to our long good-bye approaches. A tidal wave of sorrow welled up in me, attempting to drown my spirit. *Come what may, our sadness will not be the ending to Oscar's story.*

November 22nd: Today is Thanksgiving Day, a very special holiday of ours. Somehow, quite innocently, I mixed-up the dog's food bowls, and somehow put Winston's bowl into Oscar's food stand, and vice versa. Leave it to Oscar to love the game! It was because of his super-intense tail wagging that I looked more closely to see what was going on. With my focus on him, he began to eat the Hill's WD dry dog food intended for Winston, and Winston began to happily eat the Wingaling with brown rice! They made me laugh so hard! At 2 p.m., Oscar ate many pieces of fresh turkey breast, and in the evening he ate 1 can of Wingaling and 1 cup of dry dog food...Oscar slept downstairs tonight, and we left the sunroom door open and the outdoor lights on as per usual.

November 23rd: Joy of all joys!!! Winston is OK!!! The mass is a large lipoma! Our day stood still when we heard this wonderful news, and the four of us went for a three-mile walk to celebrate the beauty of the day...Both dogs hunted feverishly for Slippery Elm leaves, all to no avail... I only have one notation for Oscar's eating: two cups of Hills WD (this is Winston's dry dog food) with one can of Wingaling.

November 24th: Today was a cold, rainy day...The sunroom fountain is working again—I found a new frog spitter—the soft sound of the waterfall soothes Oscar tremendously...Eating habits continue along OK...I decided to reintroduce the B.S.S.T. product as I am eager to put more Slippery Elm in their diet. The pressure is on to find a replacement product due to the absence of fresh Slippery Elm leaves...I put drops of B.S.S.T. in each of the dogs' water bowls, but once again, after they noticed their water had changed, they completely avoided their water bowl and stopped drinking water. I must find a new remedy to replace the leaves!

Oscar and Winston needed to go outside during the night, and, while outside, I heard Oscar yelp with happy, fast barks. Deer? I wondered. I went outside to see. Yes, there they were, and Oscar was overjoyed! Both dogs paused in place, mesmerized, as the family of deer crossed through our yard and into the next. It was as if someone had said, "Be still! This is a moment of animal reverence."

Although they missed the leaves, Oscar and Winston learned that nature provided for an abundance of fascinating discoveries, even in their own back yard. They not only adapted to the change, but they developed into more because of it.

❧ *Gravizon From the Amazon*

November 25th: Oscar's morning feeding was an Asiago bagel with some dry dog food plus his supplements...I found Slippery Elm in powdered form at the health food store today, and tried to sprinkle it on the underside of the chicken thighs in Smothered Comfort...I wondered if this would this work as a substitute? I feel great pressure to fill in the void. Cold, rainy weather continues.

November 26th: With the weather working against us, along with the absence of fresh Slippery Elm leaves, I wanted to bring some fun into Oscar's life; I decided to introduce a new food with an irresistible aroma to keep Oscar motivated. In the morning, he ate a few nibbles of dry dog food plus his supplements and cookies. Then, at noon, he had his first feeding of homemade roasted orange chicken. We think Oscar has a sweet tooth! He absolutely loved the orange chicken! That afternoon, I continued to research online regarding other cancer-reducing remedies. The following information was learned from http://patrickkoh.com/healthwellnessblog/health-sciences-institute:

This health blog featured an article, "The Graviola Tree-Miraculous Secret," that was taken from an e-mail by Health Services Institute. I was fascinated in reading about the miraculous Graviola tree that grows deep within the Amazon Rainforest in Brazil. Its scientific name is Annona muricata, and it is known by the Spanish as Guanabana, the Portugese as Graviola, the Filipinos as Guyabanao, the Indonesians as Sirsak, the Dutch as Zuur zak and the Malaysians refer to it as Durian belanda. The fruit from the Graviola tree is slightly acidic when ripened.

Historically, the Graviola tree has been harvested by the indigenous Native Indians of South America as the bark leaves, roots, fruit and the seeds of the fruit, were used for centuries by medicine men to treat heart disease, asthma, liver problems and arthritis. Interestingly, the tales of miraculous healing drew the attention of one of America's largest drug companies that conducted more than 20 laboratory tests on the tree's anti-cancer capabilities (beginning in the 1970's).

Test results indicated that extracts from the Graviola tree were able to "effectively target and kill malignant cells in 12 types of cancer, including colon, breast, prostate, lung and pancreatic cancer. The tree compounds proved to be up to 10,000 times stronger in slowing the growth of cancer cells than Adriamycin, a commonly used chemotherapy drug. Unlike chemotherapy, the compound extracted from the Graviola tree selectively hunts down and kills only cancer cells. It does not harm healthy cells!"

As the Graviola tree is a natural product, federal law prohibits any such patenting which diminished the billion-dollar drug company's hopes of huge profits. They were not completely deterred. Rather, they began a seven-year research project in hopes of developing the capability of synthesizing two of the Graviola tree's most potent anti-cancer properties. What they learned, though, was that the natural properties could not be replicated. With enormous financial gain no longer a possibility, the company discontinued the research project and did not publish its findings. What a missed opportunity to benefit humanity!

However, one scientist from the Graviola tree research project did not allow this to be the end of the story. He understood the human value of the research project. Risking his career, he contacted a company that was dedicated to harvesting medicinal plants with a mission of social responsibility from the Amazon Rainforest, and shared what had been learned.

I found it interesting that the National Cancer Institute had been the first to perform a scientific study on the Graviola tree's effectiveness, yielding results that indicated Graviola's "leaves and stems were found effective in attacking and destroying malignant cells." Laboratory data from 20 other independent studies were conducted regarding the viability of Graviola, and yet no benchmark double-blind clinical trials were ever initiated. Coming from a perspective that believes in and promotes goodwill to all, this truth was a disturbing reality for me.

A study conducted at Catholic University of South Korea yielded data showing one chemical in Graviola was found to "selectively kill colon cancer cells at 10,000 times the potency of Adriamycin".... "Graviola was shown to selectively target the cancer cells, leaving healthy cells untouched." A study at Purdue University yielded data indicating "that leaves from the Graviola tree killed cancer cells among six human cell lines and were especially effective against prostrate, pancreatic and lung cancers... (http://patrickkkoh.com/healthNwellnessblog/health-sciences-institute)."

I had discovered our next product! I decided to order Gravizon supplements (rather than graviola tree in its liquid form due to our earlier experience with B.S.S.T.) from www.amazonherbs.net. I admired the Amazon Herb Company for responsibly farming the rainforest, and offering its unwavering support of the native indigent tribes of the Amazon. Their actions spoke clearly to my heart. This was a beautiful, win-win moment, and I greatly anticipated the arrival of this fascinating product the next morning via overnight mail.

November 27th: What an excellent day! The Gravizon capsules arrived via overnight mail, and I administered the human dose to Oscar. Amazingly, he ate well today, we took our three-mile walk and everyone had a great night's sleep—including Oscar. This is the first night in ages that Oscar didn't have to go out, and he stayed in our bedroom all night long.

November 28th: Another great day! Oscar drank an entire bowl of fresh water in the morning, and had two cups of dry dog food with cut-up ham slices plus his supplements. Similar eating continued for the entire day.

November 30th: Yet another day to feel grateful...Oscar's eating pattern continues to be stable. Today, though, I received a special gift: both Oscar and Winston slept on my feet (under my desk) while I worked on a writing project. It was a moment too beautiful for words—Oscar, and even Winston, too, seem so peaceful now that we are no longer searching for something to fill the void of the leaves. Oscar's willingness to take his supplements, and present-day acceptance of having even more capsules to swallow—could he possibly feel relieved that we now have a replacement for the fresh Slippery Elm leaves? Or, maybe they want me to just sit still and to share a peaceful moment with them? The amount of time left together is uncertain, but we can savor this beautiful moment – a true gift of the present moment.

Today, they found a precious new way to show their love. Love will carry us through every season.

CHAPTER THREE

Last Winter With Oscar

❧ *The Role of Fierce Pride*

December 1st: Winter may not yet have officially arrived, but the days of snowfall, the festive decorations, the aroma of holiday baking, parties, Christmas carols being played over the radio along with the daily countdown of shopping days left until Christmas (Chanukah and Kwanzaa, too) tell me otherwise. It is nearly seven months since the date of Oscar's diagnosis, and our day began with a big smile. So-very-proud-of-himself, Oscar burst open the bedroom door this morning after, again, sleeping downstairs…We took a short walk (1½ miles) today, but upon returning home, Oscar had no appetite and very low energy. He just lay there listless, on the rug in the garage, and we cannot help but feel that his passing is near. He may be experiencing his favorite things for one last time…However, things changed when Richard came home later in the evening. Searching for Oscar, Richard found him lying on the soft rugs in the garage. Richard began his usual banter with Oscar, and, sure enough, when Richard handed the Milkbone to Oscar, he perked up and ate it! It was almost as if he did so just because of Richard's dialogue and his enormous pride feeling capable of pleasing him. Ever the gamester! We put food in his bowl, and he even got up to eat it! The rule is to *never give up:* at 9 p.m., he was ready to eat!!

December 3rd: I will be in Washington, D.C. for a few days of special events with Congressman and Dr. Mary Regula and a group from the National First Ladies' Library. *Richard's-style takes over...* Oscar's day began slowly, as frequently happens. He had an appetite pill, then his vitamin and cookies plus two slices of bread. At noon, he had two slices of bread with his supplements, but he also ate a plain ground veal sandwich from a local restaurant! His evening meal was comprised of *four cans of Wingaling!* Oscar and Winston did some playing and sniffing together today, and Winston acted out by expressing his dominance and alpha dog nature. As careful as I'm sure that Richard was to disguise the special treatment to Oscar, Winston may sense an imbalance in the treats. What is one to do?

The next few days were filled with many fun moments for Richard and Oscar. Richard brought home special chicken and veal parmesan sandwiches for Oscar's lunch and he devoured them! Their practiced routine —Oscar dashing through the doggy door the instant he heard the garage door opener activate—their secret meeting in the third garage where Richard would unwrap the surprise. Oscar would wait ever so patiently as Richard blew on each piece of the sandwich to ensure the correct temperature for Oscar's eating...feeding him one bite at a time; such an act of caring from Richard to Oscar. Meanwhile, Mr. Winston waited patiently inside for his very own treat (one or two small pieces) from Richard.

December 8th: Oscar did not require the appetite medicine today. He had two steak rolls today, and played a "keep away" food game with

Winston. This may be in retaliation to Winston's dominance from the other evening. They are back to competing again!

December 9th: Today began as a very poor eating day. In the evening, the dogs came over to me to go for a walk, and it was an especially interesting one. Winston cut it short at 2½ miles as he spotted a ground hog moving in the other direction. We let him lead the way home! Oscar's appetite was tremendous this evening! If nothing else works I try to make orange chicken for him! Richard loves to feed Oscar orange chicken, too.

December 10th: In the morning, Oscar carried a steak roll in his mouth as he paraded all over the backyard, and walked up the hill to eat it. He also ate last evening's salmon leftovers. Late afternoon, Oscar came into the kitchen and looked at me in that special way as if to say, "What are you cooking tonight?" So, I made him four salmon burgers and he loved the aroma. He ate one, savoring each bite, and then went outside to take a nap in the snow!! The day went along very well, and Oscar also had a very good evening, choosing to sleep with us upstairs.

Oscar was very interested in affiliating with us today. It appeared to be so real and authentic that it seemed permanent, but the voice of hesitation resounds in my thoughts. Dare I say that our circumstances are better?

❧ The Dark Surprise

December 11th: This day began routinely, but it did not end so. On

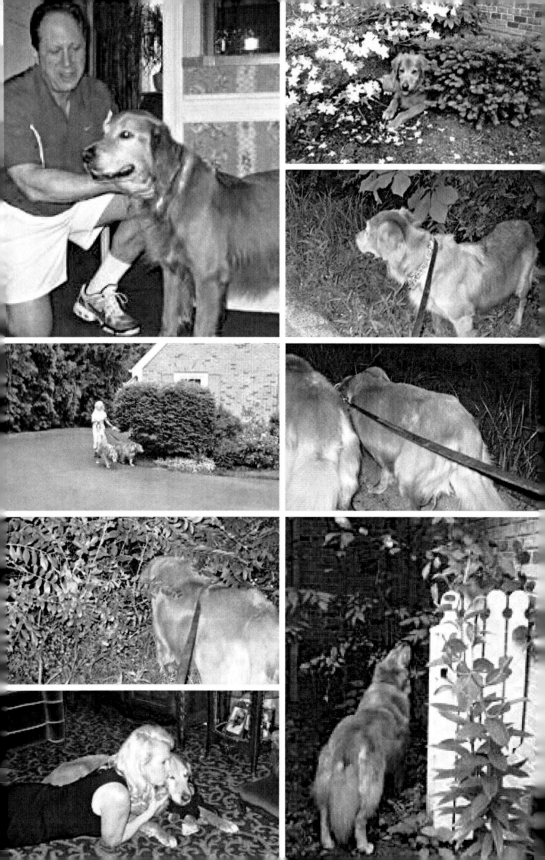

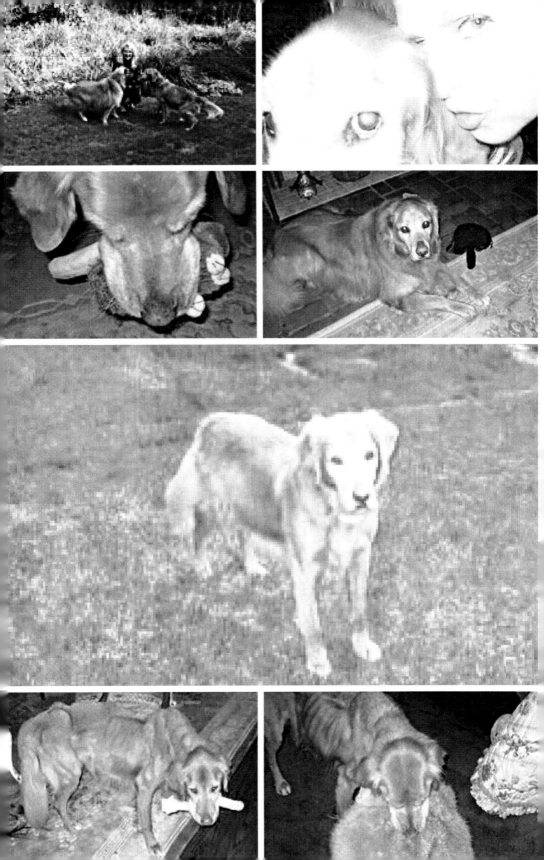

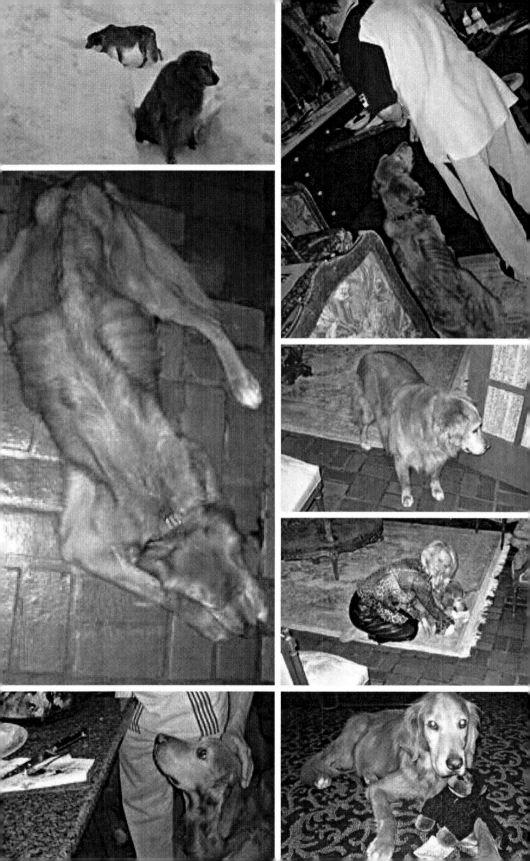

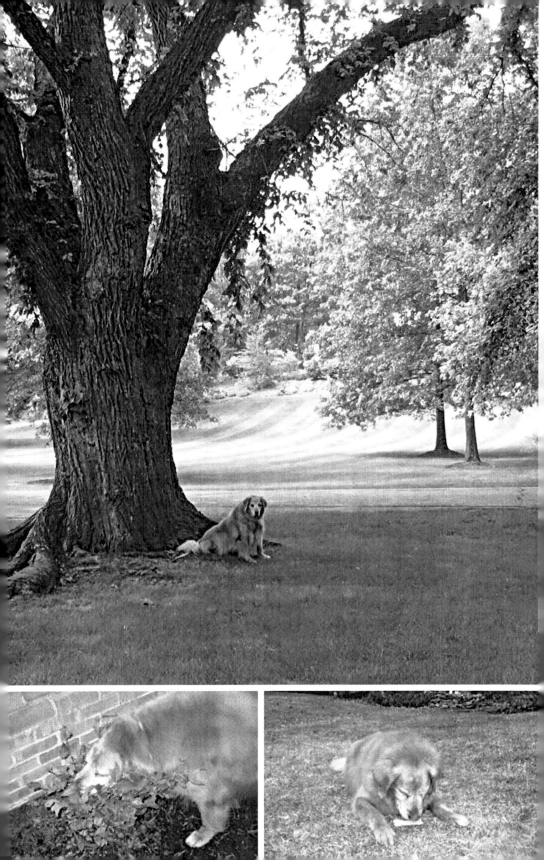

the contrary, our evening events were jolted by a very dark surprise.

Shortly after 9 p.m., the dogs approached me for a walk. I grabbed my coat and off we went, turning left at the end of our driveway, and making two more lefts at the next two intersections. All of a sudden, I felt a blast of cold air coming from my left and I sensed danger! Out of the darkness sprang two animals! I was holding Winston's leash with my left hand and Oscar's with my right. The animals, two boxers, sprang at us like predators—both began to attack Winston and I broke between them, knocking one of the dogs off Winston with my right knee. The other dog was preparing to kill his prey and had grasped Winston by his neck. Poor Winston was terrified as he tried to fight back and wrestle free. My efforts to knock this dog off of Winston while holding onto Oscar were futile. I screamed out for the neighbor who owned the dogs! "Your dog is killing my dog!!" One neighbor from across the street came running out, then the owner came out from his house, too — he made attempts to get control of his dog, but nothing worked. Meanwhile, the menacing animal was rocking Winston's neck back and forth, and I realized there were only seconds left to Winston's life!! *Loudly, ever so loudly, I began to pray, "Father God, send your mighty angels to protect Winston. Help us to know what to do!!"*

In that instant, all noise and movement ceased. The boxer stopped rocking Winston's neck back and forth. Time stood still. Without a second's pause, I stepped next to my neighbor who was kneeling beside his boxer. Placing myself in a position of dominance, I swung my leg over the boxer to straddle him. I quickly placed my gloved hands into its mouth, positioning my fingers between his teeth. I refused to let this savage dog destroy Winston! With borrowed strength, I pried his teeth apart and opened his mouth to free Winston. Winston was freed, but his face remained inches away from the face of his attacker. I held the end of Winston's leash in my left hand, and carefully began to walk away assuming he would follow. He did not.

The neighbor kept holding onto his dog, but neither of us was aware that he was also holding onto Winston's collar. I called for Winston to come to me as I began to walk from the crowd. I still had Oscar on a leash with my right hand, and needed to protect him, too! But, Winston sat there erect and motionless, his head inches away from the boxer. I had to get him out of there! I yelled louder and more frantically as everyone kept on watching.

Finally, our neighbor realized that he was holding onto part of Winston's collar, released him, and our beloved Winston began to walk toward me!! The neighbors watching wanted to cheer! All I wanted to do was to get away to a place of safety before anything else happened. I quickly walked Oscar and Winston away into the darkness where we wouldn't be seen. Feeling safe, I quickly turned to Winston who had begun to shake all over, and hugged him close while trying to reassure him as I monitored Oscar's reaction. Had Oscar been attacked, he would have been killed due to his physical condition. How thankful I was for what did *not* happen! We cuddled there together for a few minutes to regroup from the terrible scare.

One of the neighbors that had witnessed the attack drove by us, and offered some kind words. Then, the police car arrived, but there was nothing the officer could do now. We slowly began to walk the short distance home. When we got home, we found Richard on the phone. The neighbor responsible for the boxers had already phoned to apologize for the incident. Richard thoroughly examined Winston. Remarkably, his injuries were minor compared to what he had been through. I will call Dr. Heller in the morning.

December 12th: Oscar was up vomiting at 5 a.m. Somehow, though, he just didn't seem to be that sick. Then, when I gave him his supplements, I noticed something amazing. Oscar's gums were a brighter, deeper hue of pink! This was the first such day of observable progress! What a gift this was, and what a perfect morning for the discovery.

My call to Dr. Heller's office resulted in an immediate trip over to the Animal Care Clinic with Winston. Dr. Heller's compassionate response was greatly appreciated. "This dog is very lucky to be alive!" he said. Winston was going to be OK, but he would need to spend the night with them. We would be able to pick him up tomorrow morning. Funny, but when I returned home, I found Oscar lying on his back "sunning" himself on the grass in front of the sunroom door. Silly dog, Oscar!! It wasn't a sick day after all!

December 13th: I picked up Winston at 8:30 this morning, and he seems to be doing OK. With all that he experienced, we wanted to be certain he received extra love. Unfortunately, Oscar surprised us by offering a most unusual greeting upon Winston's return home. When Winston and I walked in the back door, Oscar got up from his favorite family room spot, and Winston's tail began to wag. Oscar walked closer toward Winston and then growled fiercely at him. We were surprised to see him react this way. Poor Winston! Feelings hurt, he walked off to HIS favorite spot in the room and laid down...It's easy to see how quickly jealousy and envy issues may be aroused. I reprimanded Oscar, he laid down, and then I made sure they both got the same amount of petting. This always seemed to resolve their issues when they were puppies.

December 14th: This was a poor eating day for Oscar. He refused to eat any of the canned dog food. Is Winston an issue? I sense some disturbance. Could it be possible that Oscar resents Winston knowing he only has a short time left with us? Richard and I agree this is a possibility knowing how human-like Golden Retrievers can be.

December 15th: Another day of unusual behavior from Oscar. While he had his cookies and vitamin, he refused to eat any food from his dish, eating Winston's leftover food instead. He ate nothing at noon and refused any Wingalings for his p.m. feeding. It was time for *Richard's-style* to come to the rescue! When we were nearly finished with our dinner at the Black Heath restaurant, Richard asked our waitress to have the chef make a special hamburger for Oscar. We returned home eager to share the hamburger with Oscar, but didn't find him at any of his usual places. That little gamester had somehow managed to sneak out the sunroom doggy door before we left for dinner (how he did this required some carefully planned strategy). There he was, all curled up in the sunroom with snow covering him! I was grateful to find him, but struggled with the issue of his mischief. How does one reprimand a dying dog such as our Oscar? He'd been out in the snow playing with the guys shoveling our walk while we were gone! What was his issue?....

Was he angry with us? Or, with Winston? I couldn't bear for him to feel left out...All seemed to be forgotten when he met Richard in their "hideout" where he received his exceptional surprise. He quickly ate the huge, delicious plain hamburger and offered huge kisses to his master.

December 20th: Oscar continues to be agitated. He refused any food for his a.m. feeding, but at noon he ate two large Milkbones. At 5 p.m., I brought home a present I had received from my friends, Cathy and Patrick Trumble, and placed it on one of the chairs in the family room. *It was two stuffed Golden Retriever puppies, made of real fur, in a basket.* Winston sniffed them suspiciously, checking to be certain they were not real, but Oscar appeared disinterested. However, when we returned home from dinner, I discovered that the heads had been chewed off!! I found both of the heads beside Oscar who was lying in his favorite spot in the family room....We removed the stuffed animals from the room, along with the basket, and both Richard and I spent a good amount of time tonight petting and massaging Oscar and Winston.

Oscar and Winston's capacity to love and experience emotion have surpassed our understanding. Now more aware, we will honor their sensitivities and help them to heal.

✦ Creative Feeding and the Community's Dog Food

December 22nd: Oscar's theatrics began early today. It was about 7:30 a.m. when I began to water the plants in the sunroom; Oscar was lying there watching me. I had just given him 1½ slices of Pane Turano bread and Winston had received half of a slice. As both dogs love this bread, I assumed they would begin to eat it immediately. I turned my back for a moment to gather up their dog bowls and to fill one with dry dog food for Winston. When I turned around, I looked over at them and saw that Oscar had tucked the 1 ½ slices of bread under his chin along with a couple of his stuffed toys and was just lying there on the rug acting cute. I realized he was showing off his amazing skills to merit more attention, and I began to laugh at his cuteness…He happily got up and came over to me as I was filling his bowl with Nutastics. Pronto! He reached into the bowl and began to devour the Nutastics, and ate about 95% of the bowl. It was Oscar at his silliest, and he knew I loved to see him create these scenarios. This was between us, and Winston felt quite left out; he huffed and puffed and arched his back until I came over to fuss over him, too. These dogs are too much!

It is difficult to have a ready supply of homemade foods for Oscar after the long stretch of meeting his needs. We resolved to put our energy into the activities that yield the most happiness and increased health for Oscar. Our outreach for foods that are a good source of protein and also a flavor that appeals to him has now led us to many of our surrounding restaurants and deli's. *Richard's-style*, vibrant and creative, is guaranteed to produce positive results for Oscar!

December 23rd: Oscar was up early this morning vomiting, but by 9 a.m., he was ready for his vitamin and a cookie along with an assortment of small, flavored Milkbones. I put Nutastics in his bowl at 9:30 a.m. and he ate them as if they were real dry dog food. At noon, he ate one large Milkbone plus a half dozen or so of the Three Dog

Bakery's carob sandwich cookies. The evening feeding consisted of two varieties of dry dog food plus his supplements (including Gravizon) followed by several carob sandwich cookies...

December 24th (Christmas Eve): At 8 a.m., Oscar ran outside to vomit, which meant that he had vomited up his appetite pill. This became a miracle day as he went on to eat naturally. It was a very good eating day, beginning with a breakfast of French toast, along with his dry dog food...Sadly, Winston's third attempt to nuzzle and show love to Oscar was met with stiff indifference. Oscar will not wag his tail around Winston and behaves strangely towards him. The resentment issue continues to be present.

December 25th (Christmas Day): This was a great day for both dogs, and, thankfully, Oscar had no difficulty eating. Breakfast included ricotta pancakes along with his usual supplements, and he eagerly ate a plain hamburger with the bun at noon. His evening feeding included rolls, duck and sweet potatoes placed on top of his dry dog food.

December 26th: This was an especially fun eating day for Oscar! His early morning feeding included 3 small, flavored Milkbone cookies along with his 3 morning supplements and some Nutastics. At noon, he ate a ground veal parmesan sandwich from La Pizzaria's Restaurant, and in the p.m., he a plain Chick-fil-A sandwich served *Richard's-style*. So many of our local restaurants are happily joining in our feeding efforts to keep Oscar alive! We took a 2 ¾ mile walk, the first walk since the December 11th incident. For obvious reasons, we avoided the location where the attack occurred.

December 27th: Today began slowly for Oscar. I gave him some all-natural, heart-shaped bacon cookies with his vitamin, supplements, and Gravizon capsule. At noon, he eagerly ate a plain McDonald's Quarter Pounder served *Richard's style*. A special moment of silliness with Oscar happened in the afternoon when it was time for his PhytoPharmica Cellular Forte with IP-6 & Inositol tablet. He ran from me, scooted upstairs and positioned himself at the top of the stairs with paws hanging down and panting happily—always eager to receive his supplements and to turn any routine moment into a game of great fun! This was also a good night for us as he slept through the entire night without having to go outside.

December 28th: At 7:30 a.m., I gave Oscar an appetite pill, and he and Winston began their day normally by going outside. They began to bark at something and I listened carefully. Yes! There was a big difference in Oscar's bark, and it sounded strong and almost back to normal! Variety is important to a creative dog such as Oscar, so I gave him three different dog foods, each layered over the other. He responded to the uniqueness of his feeding with spirited mischief and ate from both his own and Winston's (Winston was still outside) bowls. I removed Winston's bowl and refilled what he had eaten, and then brought Winston into the room to eat.

December 30th: Oscar had the hiccups two times today! At 2 p.m., he ate a plain Chick-fil-A sandwich, and another at 8:30 p.m. Soft chicken Milkbones cookies were Oscar's treat following each of his supplements today. He loves these, too!

December 31st: Cold winter weather remains a constant. Unfortunately, the weather forecasters are predicting a harsh winter in Northeast Ohio. Eating pattern continues. For his p.m. feeding, Oscar ate a whole ground veal parmesan sandwich along with an assortment of cookies and his supplements.

January 1st: Happy New Year! The morning ritual of having a dog vitamin along with with dog treat continues for Oscar and Winston. Today, though, Oscar ate only his vitamin!? He ate a nice portion of French toast made with Pane Turano bread for his morning feeding, and around 1 p.m., he surprised us by eating 1 ½ ground veal parmesan sandwiches with bun. Richard sensed he was able to eat more today, so at 2 p.m., he offered Oscar the remaining two plain Chick-fil-A's we had in the fridge. He ate it all! Apparently energized, he dashed out through the doggy door and entered the third garage "hideout" where he had hidden his large rawhide bone. At 3:30 p.m., he was still happily entertained in the backyard and appeared to be relaxing out there, completely focused on chewing. Winston was outside with him, too.

January 6th: We had an 8 a.m. wake-up from Oscar—his licks on our faces were such a great start to the day! Because he refused to eat his vitamin and cookie, I gave him an appetite pill. At 10 a.m., he came into the kitchen where I was working so I gave him some pieces of his favorite French toast, but he was only able to eat 6-7 pieces. At 11:30 a.m., he came into the kitchen again and stood there watching me. I enthusiastically responded, thinking he was up to another game. Sure enough! He dashed outside and lay right in front of the kitchen window where I could see him. Once I noticed him there, he responded with a very focused watch on me. It was another moment of deep connection for us! Shortly after noon, he was able to eat two plain Chick-fil-A sandwiches. There is no doubt in my mind that he is still having a quality life despite his very thin physique.

January 7th: We see notable progress! Oscar continues to be able to eat and is also able to chew rawhides. Both dogs have loved rawhides since they were puppies, so it is wonderful for him to consistently be able to enjoy this fun tradition. His tongue and gums are a much brighter pink, but now there is a large growth under his tongue...We took a 2 ½ mile walk today, again avoiding the back loop.

January 8th: At noon today, Oscar ate half of a veal parmesan sandwich. The p.m. feeding was interesting as Oscar refused Wingalings and another veal parmesan sandwich. He responded to the two plain double hamburgers I brought home from Wendy's. When he stopped eating the second hamburger, I played a game with him! I tried a small piece, and as I began to chew he reached out to eat more!

January 9th: Oscar was funny at breakfast today. He ate nearly an entire asiago bagel, but only if we BOTH fed him the pieces! This was a powerful moment of shared love between us, and Winston was given his share of pieces, too. At 4:30 p.m., he was able to eat ¾ of a grilled hamburger (without salt) from the Black Heath restaurant along with plenty of soft Milkbones chicken cookies with his supplements...Around 9 p.m. or so, he drank a tremendous amount of water from his bowl and appeared to be hungry again. He was able to eat ¾ of another grilled hamburger and 6 ½ carob sandwich cookies with his supplements...We took a 2½ mile walk this evening. Amazingly, Oscar was eager for his walk and did superbly.

January 13th: We introduced Oscar to bacon over the past few days, and he is quite excited when Richard heads out to Perkins in the early morning, and then returns home to feed him one strip at a time. At noon, Oscar responded to soft Milkbones chicken cookies and his p.m. feeding consisted of almost an entire veal parmesan sandwich on top of his dry dog food. The growth in his mouth is definitely affecting his eating, and Richard is contemplating whether or not he should remove it. He ate many soft Milkbones chicken cookies with his supplements this evening.

January 14th: This was a sad day on the journey. The dogs had their bath and grooming appointments today, but this one will be Oscar's last appointment. Their groomer, Lisa, mentioned that even the bath has become too much for him. This brings a gripping wave of sorrow into my heart as I absorb the meaning of the loss. We are walking the journey of a slow and gentle good bye. It is difficult to imagine taking Winston to Oak Shadows by himself, leaving Oscar at home…alone.

These moments are opportunities to practice courage. We will measure up to whatever we are expected to do.

❧ Red Clover

January 16th: This was a very poor eating day. Oscar ate three large

Milkbones in the a.m., but was disinterested in food the remainder of the day. We feel that he is able to eat, but that the growing tumor in his mouth has complicated the issue.

January 17th: This, too, was a slow eating day. The tumor under Oscar's tongue is majorly interfering with his ability to eat. Once again, I felt a great urging to address the issue with another natural remedy. I discussed the situation with Marcia Vahila, an accomplished massotherapist. She immediately thought of red clover as it is good for circulation. I will begin to research its usefulness for Oscar. I will also switch foods again to see what will interest him...We reintroduced rice today and built upon Oscar's current fondness of bacon. He was able to eat a small bowl of rice with bacon in the a.m. He refused all attempts to interest him in eating at noon, and we have much concern. At 5:30 p.m., Oscar reacted positively to cut-up pieces of fresh chicken breast and ate an entire breast with a small amount of rice. At 9 p.m., Richard offered Oscar three large Milkbones, and he ate them all. His love of the soft chicken flavored Milkbones continues, and as far as we're concerned, he can have as many as he wants before falling asleep! Once the dogs were upstairs for the evening, I turned on my computer to learn about red clover.

As with Slippery Elm and Graviola tree extract, I learned that red clover, also known as Trifolium pratense, is well known to medical science. According to the University of Maryland Medical Center, "Red clover is a wild plant that is used for grazing cattle and other animals. It has also been used medicinally to treat a number of conditions. Traditionally, these have included cancer, whooping cough, respiratory problems, and skin inflammations, such as psoriasis and eczema. Red clover was thought to "purify" the blood by acting as a diuretic (helping the body get rid of excess fluid) and expectorant (helping clear lungs of mucous), improving circulation, and helping cleanse the liver." Additionally, "researchers have begun to study isoflavones from red clover. There is some preliminary evidence that they may stop cancer cells from growing or kill cancer cells in test tubes (www.umm.edu/altmed/articles/red-clover-000270.htm)." The website listed 24 supporting research studies.

According to www.herbwisdom.com, red clover is known to be a rich source of isoflavones which are water-soluble chemicals that act like estrogens and are found in many plants. Further, red clover is a good source of many essential nutrients such as calcium, chromium, magnesium, niacin, phosphorus, potassium, thiamine, and vitamin C. Red clover is "indicated for preventing endometrial cancer in women and limiting prostate cancer in men."

There were echoes of praise for the sweet herb. "It is a component of several well-known herbal formulas including some formulas of Essiac tea and various herbalist's formulas and combinations...Due to its anti-cancer activity, red clover poultices are also used on cancerous growths visible on the surface of the body (www.all4naturalhealth.com/red-clover-benefits.html)."

Red clover was our next remedy! It was available at a local health food store, and I planned to buy some tomorrow morning.

January 18th: My early morning visit to the health food store was very productive. In addition to purchasing red clover in capsule form, I also found an excellent new dry dog food for both dogs to try! It would be wonderful to have them both eat the same thing...Once home, Oscar was at my side when I put the new dog food into his bowl. Because he was so interested, I put several cups of food in his bowl. It was astonishing! He ate all of the food in his bowl — I interrupted him three times to give him his two capsules of red clover and the Gravizon supplement, but he resumed eating after each interruption…There was no finicky attitude about eating or not eating! As with the addition of Gravizon, Oscar seemed relieved that there was a remedy for his current issue. His mood change was obvious to us — he was happy and proud of himself and his ability to eat!! After dinner, he followed me to my office, and remained cozily with me the entire evening! It's such a wonderful feeling to again be in sync with his needs.

January 19th: The effectiveness of red clover was apparent this morning! I couldn't believe my eyes—in just one day, the edges of the tumor had already turned from red to the color of Oscar's tongue…Oscar ate seven small flavored Milkbones with his morning supplements plus four slices of bacon. At 3:15 p.m., he ate ¾ of a plain Chick-fil-A, plus five all-natural bacon (heart) cookies. At 5:30 p.m., he ate two cups of his new dog food plus his capsules of red clover and Gravizon.

January 20th: Oscar's a.m. feeding consisted of nibbles of dry dog food and his supplements. At noon he ate soft Milkbones chicken cookies with his supplements, and at 5 p.m., he ate very well: a bowl of dry dog food with more soft chicken cookies on top plus his supplements.

January 21st: A heavy snowstorm hit Northeast Ohio today. Both dogs had fun eating snow today, and I noticed that Oscar ate the snow in lieu of drinking his water.

January 22nd: Oscar was hungry this morning, and he readily ate dry dog food with some soft Milkbones chicken cookies plus his supplements. Red clover's effect continues to be obvious on the tumor. In just four days, the bright red color is gone, and the existing color of the entire tumor is now a medium hue of pink. In the evening, he ate his dog food with a large portion of mashed sweet potatoes on top with his supplements. During the day, Oscar had a large plain rawhide and Winston had a beef basted rawhide. Oscar also ate 2 large Milkbones, 10 soft chicken Milkbones cookies and also some pieces of orange chicken.

January 24th: The day began slowly for Oscar, and I believe that last night's walk overly fatigued him. He has such pride and inner strength—we admire him so much for his ability to persevere. How a dog in his condition could possibly walk so far in the snow is beyond our understanding...At noon, he chose bites of turkey over bread and readily ate real bacon cookies in the afternoon. At 6 p.m., Oscar ate ¼ plain hamburger with the bun plus his supplements. At 9:30 p.m., he appeared able to eat, and we fed him the remaining ¾ of the hamburger plus two supplements...Both dogs headed upstairs to their beds, and I followed with their treats. However, Oscar snuck out of the bedroom when I was distracted, and as I was searching for him, I heard Richard's voice coming from downstairs. Curious, I went down to see what they were up to. Oscar was lying beside Richard watching a great tennis match! When they came upstairs later, Oscar had six soft chicken Milkbones cookies and some orange chicken.

January 25th: Today was an extremely cold day. Oscar and Winston have always loved the cold and the snow, but we always have limited their exposure for obvious reasons. Oscar climbed the back hill this morning, and I watched him carefully to keep close tabs on him. Lately, I sense he is defying his good judgment just to be able to do things one more time. Sure enough, once he got to the top of the hill, he held his paw up which indicated how cold he was. I immediately rushed out to him to rub his paws, and urged him to come in with Winston. His face was so terribly sad, so strikingly sad. He walked very slowly down the hill with me. This was another heart-wrenching moment that I could only hope to ease by reassuring him and hugging him close. When we were inside, I covered him with his soft blue blanket, and he curled up to sleep. Winston was nearby all covered up and doing the same…Oscar only ate ½ plain Quarter Pounder plus one large Milkbones cookie today, and this was at noon.

January 26th: Today was a better day for us. Oscar ate 10 cut-up pieces of French toast in the morning, two of which came from Richard at the breakfast table. At noon, he readily ate orange chicken, and in the evening he ate a plain double hamburger. We were able to do all of his supplements today. I don't give him his supplements on the days he isn't eating very well as we don't want him to feel poorly from the remedies when there isn't enough intake of food to properly absorb the nutrients, etc.

January 27th: Oscar laid outside in the snow from approximately 9:45 a.m.-10 a.m. this morning, and then I brought him inside. He was able to eat some French toast this morning, half of a Wendy's plain double hamburger at noon, and an entire plain Quarter Pounder from McDonald's in the evening.

January 28th: What about feeding Oscar baby food? Friends have suggested baby food to me many times over the past months as another option. Today, I offered Oscar varieties of baby food today, but he was disinterested. We make every effort to respect his inability to eat, but he is so weak from not eating.... Today, I whistled for Oscar and Winston to come join me as I was reading on the loveseat by the window upstairs. This has always been a favorite resting activity for them, and they would compete to see who got to sit closest to me. I tried to spark Oscar's interest by this activity! Weak and wobbly, and with our help, he made it up the stairs to lie beside me and rested well. Amazingly, he walked down and up again later that evening and curled up beside my side of the bed for the night.

January 30th: Today, Oscar ate ground veal with some rice for his a.m. and noon feedings. In the evening when I was making a fresh batch, I decided to leave the veal in big chunks whenever possible as Oscar continues to respond to protein. Silly Oscar! He noticed the difference in the size of the veal, and responded with enthusiastic eating! I found some new carob chip dog cookies today, and he ate many cookies while resting on his bed tonight. For every full cookie that Oscar gets, Winston gets a piece of one.

January 31st: The tumor is disappearing!! It is much smaller in size! Oscar was able to eat ground veal and rice at all of his feedings today. Red clover is working beautifully!

February 1st: At 8:30 a.m., Oscar ate ⅔ piece of Pane Turano bread toasted with three of his supplements. Silly Oscar stole Winston's rawhide at 10:30 a.m., and dashed out the doggy door to eat it outside in the rain. Winston just stared at him from the window (unless someone holds the doggy door open for him, Winston is unable to use it). I intervened in the issue and brought Oscar inside, giving them each a new rawhide, but gave Winston's back to him. They seemed satisfied with the intervention. Before I left at 11 this morning, I decided to brush their teeth, which in the past, usually created somewhat of a stir in Oscar. I began with Winston, who has always loved this activity, and then I proceeded to prepare Oscar's toothbrush. I laid the toothbrush aside, and gathered up Oscar's favorite blanket and toys, and nestled them around him. The blanket has always brought him comfort, and it did so again. He allowed me to quickly brush his teeth! In the evening, Oscar nibbled at the ground veal and ate two large Milkbones.

I explored www.onlynatural pet.com/product Web site for additional remedies, hoping to find other products that addressed Oscar's needs. I discovered Cellullar Forte Max3, a clinically researched product that provides triple strength support to boost natural killer cell and immune system activity. This product was essentially three times stronger than PhytoPharmica Cellular Forte with IP-6 & Inositol. Oscar needed all the help we could give him! I placed an order and requested next day delivery.

February 2nd: I gave Oscar an appetite pill this morning. Around 10:30-11 a.m., he ate two large Milkbones along with the tablets of Cellular Forte Max3 which had just arrived. He was right beside me when the box arrived and watched closely as I unpacked the box. The most natural thing for me to do was to give him his newest supplement!

At noon, he was disinterested in everything I offered him, including a Chick-fil-A. At 1 p.m., he walked toward me, and I could tell he was communicating his interest in eating something. He ate a full cup of ground veal with some rice, and then went outside to nap. Interestingly, he came back inside somewhat later and walked toward me again. I prepared more veal with rice, and filled his large bowl completely with the mixture. He eagerly ate it all and four heaping mounds of sweet potatoes, too! *Our beloved Oscar has learned so many effective ways to communicate with us.*

February 3rd: This was a day that tugged on our heartstrings. Oscar was unable to eat anything all day. Or, so it seemed! At 4 p.m., Oscar walked toward me, indicating that he wanted to go for a walk. I prepared myself for the necessity of taking a short walk to the park and back. As we approached the park, Oscar indicated his awareness of my thoughts and crossed behind me, announcing we were not turning around, but walking, at least to the next road (this would make the walk slightly more than a mile long). He kept this pattern up for the entire walk and when the Village police car passed us, the kind lady officer cheered Oscar on! We walked 2 ½ miles!

His want to communicate with us. His strength. His conviction. I was so moved and inspired by Oscar that I went to work immediately to make him his favorite orange chicken when we returned home. Nothing was more important than rewarding him for this moment. This frail dog, whose appearance was likened to skeletal images of animals that endured years of famine, was teaching us how to live!

At 8 p.m., Oscar ate nearly a whole orange chicken. We couldn't feed it to him fast enough!

It is gratifying to watch Richard feed it to him!

February 4th: Oscar began his day by eating two large Milkbones along with his supplements. In the evening, he ate ¾ cup dog food with ¾ cup orange chicken. He took his remaining supplement with a large slice of Pane Turano bread.

February 5th: This was a non-eating day. Oscar drank lots of water, but he refused any and all foods and treats that we offered him. We kept our spirits up, and did not focus on any negativity. Oscar is very weak today, and we responded with gentleness and love.

February 6th: Today was a better day. Oscar is walking much better, and he spent time hunting outside and interacting with Winston. We gave him an appetite pill in the morning, and at noon I found him lying on his favorite strip of ground by the garage. It was just wide enough for him to rest easily in it. Silly Oscar! He came inside, and was able to eat one large Milkbones cookie and 13 soft chicken Milkbones cookies. At 4 p.m., Richard brought him a plain Chick-fil-A sandwich, and he ate nearly all of it. Later in the evening, he ate 1 large Milkbones cookie and four big pieces of rotisserie chicken.

February 7th: Oscar had fun with the people in our home today. Everyone was trying to give him food, and it turned into a game for him! He was given a large Milkbones cookie from Janet, and responded well to Crystal's nurturing. Seeing him perched at the top of the stairs, she approached him with respect and dignity. He listened to her words, then looked up at her and ate the two small Milkbones and the vitamin she left him. The stories others share with us about how he interacts with them are heartwarming. Oscar saw me by the cupboard (where their dog treats are kept) and walked toward me. I focused on his communication, and then decided he wanted more Nutastics put in his bowl, so I took out the container and walked over to his bowl with him. His tail wagged at his achievement! Richard and I find his new communication process to be so much fun. In the evening, he ate ¾ of a plain double hamburger. He ate another 20 of the peanut butter Nutastics thanks to the work of everyone! We are encouraged by all of his socializing. So is Winston! I also sense that Oscar really enjoys listening to music when he rests in the family room. Both dogs just lay still as they listened to mellow and energizing music.

February 8th: This was an excellent morning. Oscar was able to happily eat many pieces of French toast made with Pane Turano bread, and several pieces of Richard's asiago bagel. Of course, Winston had some, too. At noon, Oscar ate an entire plain double hamburger from Wendy's.

February 9th: Oscar is radiating joy and a beautiful energy! This was a complete WOW day. His eclectic "community dog food" eating pattern has produced many supporters and fans! Every place we go to get his meal, they ask about him and wish him the best...Richard was filled with enormous joy in response to Oscar's strong physical presence and progress (Cellular Forte Max3 must be working along with the red clover and the Gravizon, etc.), but we are afraid to trust it...*During my prayers with the dogs tonight, I imagined praying from their perspective*—a prayer of thanks for the things they like. The following spontaneous prayer elicited so many licks from Oscar and Winston that I decided to write it down to preserve the moment in my memory:

"Praise to the God of all the hills, mountains and valleys; Praise to the God of all children (furry or not) and their families; Praise God from whom all blessings flow; Praise to God, the most wonderful Father who watches over us all."

My heart is completely open to this experience. May Richard and I be forever grateful for this journey.

The Heart Bowl

February 10th: Today marks nine months since Oscar's diagnosis. Tomorrow, I am hosting a retreat for the staff of the National First Ladies' Library here at our home. My treasured friend, Founder and President of the National First Ladies' Library, Mary Regula, will also be joining us. These past few days have been extremely busy with the fun of cooking and baking, and working on all of the details. Oscar's eating pattern today was similar to the days previously recorded...*Richard's style of nurturing Oscar and Winston is so helpful to me, and they love the extras he gives them.*

February 11th: The day dawned sunny and the sky is pretty, but it is very cold outside. Winston thrived on all the activities with the guests today, but Oscar withdrew from interacting with the people and laid, instead, in the sunshine of every room we were in. It was good to be able to watch him, and I found it quite comforting to see how he maximized his time in the sun. During the ladies' surprise entertainment, I sat beside him in the rear of the room, and visited with Noelle Audi-Miller. A sensitive and spiritual friend (also a minister), she understood the significance of Oscar's journey. She also offered a wonderful suggestion. Why not add vanilla Ensure to our list of food possibilities for Oscar? It had been helpful in her relative's treatment. The concept of offering liquid nutrition to Oscar sounded wonderful to me, and I bought some later that afternoon.

When I opened a bottle of Ensure, I contemplated how I could serve it to Oscar. The dog bowls were too large, and I glanced over our own bowls for something that would work. I smiled when I saw the stack of white heart bowls we used earlier in the day. Perfect! I took the top two bowls — the tiniest one would be for Winston, and the medium bowl would be for Oscar. My theory was that if I presented the new "food" enthusiastically, there would be a greater likelihood that Oscar would be receptive to it...Oscar and Winston were both lying on the carpet in the family room. I presented the vanilla Ensure as if they were getting the treat of their lifetime, and they looked at the heart bowls appreciatively. A few sniffs convinced them that this was going to be quite a novel treat, and both licked their bowls clean...Yet another way to keep Oscar going! He ate two plain Chick-fil-A sandwiches for his p.m. feeding.

February 12th: Oscar's eating today was completely voluntary, and without any appetite meds. We didn't have to feed him piece by piece, or stand by him to encourage him. This hasn't happened in the longest time! Offering Oscar a bowl of Ensure is a new game, and I was able to give him his supplements quite easily between his licks and slurps of enjoyment.

February 13th: Today's feeding schedule was the following: in the a.m., he had half a bottle of Ensure in his heart bowl with two Gravizon capsules; at 1:30 p.m., he had 1½ plain Chick-fil-A sandwiches, plus two red clover capsules; at 5:15 p.m., he had the remaining half of the Chick-fil-A with two Cellular Forte Max3 tablets. Later, he had a rawhide and many soft cookies (made with protein) to accompany his final supplements for the day.

February 14th: We are eager to get as many supplements into Oscar as is possible, but it cannot be forced. He has to be ready for the day's "work." At 9 a.m., Oscar had ⅔ of an asiago bagel with all of his morning supplements. At 11:30 a.m., he eagerly ate ¾ of a plain Chick-fil-A sandwich. Later in the afternoon, I offered him some Ensure and he drank a hearty portion from his heart bowl.

February 15th: This morning, I phoned Noelle to thank her for the very helpful suggestion! Around 10:30 a.m., Oscar had half a bottle of Ensure with his supplements. At 10:45 a.m., he went upstairs and ate his vitamin plus two small Milkbones cookies left beside his bed for him. This was the first vitamin he has eaten in a long time—such a very happy moment—and he made sure that I noticed he had eaten it! At 2:45 p.m., he was able to communicate that he was ready to eat, and I gave him 1¾ plain Chick-fil-A sandwiches plus the necessary supplements.

February 16th: This morning was very special! At 7 a.m., Oscar had his vitamin and two small Milkbones upstairs. Around 8:30 a.m., he had about five bites of an asiago bagel, and at 11:30 a.m., I offered him some fresh Ensure in his beautiful, white heart bowl. He seemed to really enjoy it and had between 40-50 licks of Ensure before he was full. At 1:45 p.m., Oscar ate two Chick-fil-A sandwiches (minus a couple of mouthfuls he left behind). Around 5:30 p.m., Richard brought home a plain double hamburger from Wendy's that he ate with his supplements... The weather continues to be very cold and snowy.

February 17th: Oscar ate his vitamin and two small Milkbones a little after 8 a.m. this morning. He had 73 slurps of Ensure at 10 a.m. with his Gravizon capsule. Amazing! At 1 p.m., he had a plain Chick-fil-A with his supplements. Then at 6 p.m., he approached me for a walk. The weather was less cold today, and the sky was clear and quite beautiful. We did the mile and a third loop, and when we returned home, Richard had a fresh double hamburger ready for Oscar. He devoured it and we were able to give him his remaining supplements. At 9 p.m., he ate half of another double hamburger.

February 18th: Oscar ate 1½ Chick-fil-A, plus his supplements, today at around 12:30 p.m. He still has not regained any interest in the dry dog food or the canned gourmet food, so we are grateful that he will get some calories this way. At 6:30 p.m., he ate a complete half pound plain, unsalted hamburger with his supplements. I have also added Slippery Elm capsules to his treatment plan. I was so pleased to discover that our health food store now carried it in capsule form! At 8:15 p.m., he ate six more pieces of a thick hamburger, plus four more supplements. Then, at bedtime, he had several small, flavored Milkbones cookies.

February 19th: This was an exceptionally cold winter day. At 6:30 a.m., he ate his vitamin and two small Milkbones, and by 10:30 a.m., he was able to enjoy nearly ⅔ a bottle of Ensure. He and Winston curled up in the family room, and I put on some gentle music. At 2 p.m., he ate 1½ Chick-fil-A, plus all of his supplements. As the day progressed, Oscar seemed to be feeling edgy due to the extra strain of the frigid weather. Richard returned home around 6:30 p.m. with a double hamburger for Oscar, but the restaurant made an error and put cheese on it. Oscar sniffed it, rejected it and came back in the house. Richard went back out to bring back another hamburger as specified, but Oscar had lost his enthusiasm and only ate half of it with four supplements. At bedtime, Oscar happily ate seven King Louis peanut butter cookies with his remaining supplements.

February 20th: At 7 a.m., Oscar ate his vitamin with two small Milkbones and was able to eat one cup of dry dog food at 8 a.m.! Wonderful! At 9:30 a.m., he had half a bottle of Ensure in his white heart bowl. At noon, he had 2½ portions of rice with ground veal plus supplements and many slurps of Ensure! This was amazing for me to see. Richard came home a little past 9 p.m. with a plain hamburger—at first, Oscar pretended to be disinterested, but with a little competition from Winston, he was able to eat a portion of it. King Louis cookies continue to be a hit, and he had six of them at bedtime with his remaining supplements.

February 22nd: Oscar woke me very early this morning with licks and tail wags! I fussed over him in return, but then fell back sound asleep. He gave me a few minutes to sleep, and then woke me all over again. Silly dog, Oscar! The day was an irregular eating day. At 8 a.m., he ate his vitamin and two small Milkbones cookies, and around 9 a.m., he had about ⅓ bottle of Ensure with his Gravizon. The snowstorms and icy weather have wrecked havoc with our security system, and the alarm problem continued until 3:30 p.m. Unfortunately, Oscar was shaken-up by the noise and chaos, and ate only a few bites of Chick-fil-A at noon, refused rice with salmon, etc. At 9 p.m., he gobbled up a bowl of Nutastics.

It is more than nine months since Oscar's diagnosis. It's time to determine which remedies are working effectively.

➷ Our Effective Combination of Remedies

February 23rd: At 6:45 a.m., Oscar ate his vitamin and a small Milkbones cookie. At 9:30 a.m., he had some Ensure and at noon nearly ¾ of a Chick-fil-A, but was disinterested in eating in the evening. I have decided to review all of his supplements and remedies, and want our decisions regarding what remains and what doesn't to be made with great precision.

February 24th: There was no interest in eating today until I pulled a portabella mushroom and goat cheese breakfast pizza from the oven! Oscar communicated that he was ready to eat, and we cautiously gave him some of the pizza. He ate it eagerly! Also, there were nibbles of an asiago bagel that we coordinated with four supplements. In the evening, I offered him dry dog food, and he was able to eat 1½ cups from his dog bowl. He, again, took his supplements with King Louis peanut butter cookies.

February 25th: In the a.m., Oscar had half of a heart bowl of Ensure with his Gravizon along with 10 King Louis cookies that were offered to him by workers taking care of house repairs today. It is a team effort to keep Oscar eating! At 4 p.m., he had some pieces of Chick-fil-A sandwich and then was disinterested with all of our efforts to offer him food. Later, he had some Ensure and more King Louis cookies with his supplements.

February 26th: Very good news! The supplements must be working as Oscar had a normal stool today. We haven't seen this since last summer.

February 27th: Oscar ate his vitamin this morning (leaving the cookies behind), but soon vomited. Later in the morning he drank nearly a full bottle of Ensure in his heart bowl, and by 4 p.m. he was able to eat a big bowl of cut-up pieces of Pane Turano bread along with chicken breast and some lamb with juices. This was a great surprise to us, and we were pleased that we were able to give him all of his supplements.

February 28th: This was a wonderful eating day! He ate well and had 3 regular meals today.

Cancer is a multi-faceted disease that must be treated with a comprehensive treatment plan. Over the past few days I have been experimenting to determine what combination of remedies is helping Oscar's current condition. The end result is that NF Spectra Probiotic, Cellular Forte Max3, Slippery Elm, red clover, Gravizon and the Only Natural Pet GI Support seem to work well together. These remedies now comprise our treatment plan. I eliminated the Only Natural Immune Strengthener and the PhytoPharmica Cellular Forte with IP-6 & Inositol as the recent additions have stronger properties.

At 8:15 a.m., he eagerly drank Ensure with his Gravizon supplement. At noon, he wanted some of Richard's pizza, and ate a half of a large piece. At 4 p.m., he ate nearly all of a plain Chick-fil-A sandwich with his supplements. Giving him cookies (without any supplements) absolutely delighted him (and Winston) at bedtime!!

March 2nd: At 8:30 this morning, Oscar had a small heart bowl of Ensure with Gravizon, and he responded to having more Ensure at 1:30 p.m., and I was able to give him his supplements. I am trying now to give him some eating and drinking time without always trying to give him supplements. Otherwise, it seems that Oscar is always "working." At 5 p.m., I prepared a huge bowl of Vienna bread (2½-3 large slices cut-up) with pieces of orange chicken with some orange sauce; he ate nearly two-thirds of the bowl!

March 4-6th: The new pattern continues nicely. Oscar is eating and he is able to eat healthy foods. He is eating his vitamin, drinking the Ensure, taking his supplements and eating nearly the entire big dog bowl of Turano bread and chicken mixture. Snowstorms continue, and the cold weather is a stressor for Oscar.

March 7th: Despite Oscar's new ability to eat, he is extremely thin and very weak. He is having trouble walking upstairs (we are now carrying him) and outside in the snow. His food intake today included his morning vitamin and cookie, dry dog food plus supplements, half of a veal parmesan sandwich with bun at noon, and a bowl of Turano bread with chicken mixture plus supplements for his evening meal. Later, at bedtime, he had Ensure with his three remaining supplements.

March 8th: The snow is now more than 2½ feet high outside, and as it was so hard for Oscar to walk in the snow to eliminate, I shoveled a walking path for the dogs to make things easier. However, Oscar's fierce pride was unrelenting—he forged through the snow creating his own path despite his frail appearance; Winston, meanwhile, appreciated the shoveled path and was happy to walk on it. I noticed him looking at his littermate in wonderment when Oscar refused to follow suit… Richard gave Oscar lobster later in the evening and he loved it! Some time later, he went outside and burrowed a path to connect with one of my "highways." He has enormous grit—Oscar, you continue to inspire us!! I captured the day's special moments in photos.

March 9th: We cannot believe that Oscar is still alive. His physical condition continues to defy the odds; the cold and the deep snow make the situation even more challenging. Unfortunately, he continued to resist walking on the shoveled "highway" and today, got stuck in the snow. I needed to shovel all around him to pull him out of the drift, and

I also shoveled a connecting path to the main path. This time, he walked the path. Winston just stood there watching us carefully...The new eating pattern has slipped. This morning, he had some French toast with his supplements. At 1:30 p.m., he had a small heart bowlful of Ensure, and by 4 p.m., he was willing to have some soft chicken Milkbones cookies. At 9 p.m., he drank nearly a full can of Ensure without any supplements.

March 10th: Today, it is 10 months since we learned of Oscar's diagnosis. This morning, he had a full can of Ensure in his heart bowl with his Gravizon and two red clover capsules. At noon, I offered him a new treat: Carver's chicken—he happily consumed four large pieces. At 6:30 p.m., he ate ¼ of a bowl of Italian bread and chicken mixture with his supplements.

March 11th: Oscar is still very weak, but today was a day of better eating. He ate six pieces of Richard's asiago bagel at breakfast (so did Winston, so I warmed another one for Richard!). Oscar laid down in the family room to drink a small amount of Ensure and had more at noon. In the late afternoon, he was able to ingest a full bottle of Ensure, and by 6 p.m., he had also eaten two strips of a plain Chick-fil-A sandwich and some dry dog food. At 9:30 p.m., he drank half of a can of Ensure with his Gravizon, two red clover and two Cellular Forte Max3. *Amazingly, at 11 p.m., Oscar rather sheepishly entered our bedroom (he walked up the stairs in the dark on his own), drank nearly ¾ of the water in the bowl and then proceeded to come over to my side of the bed to sleep. Blessings to you, Oscar!*

March 12th: At 8 a.m. today, Oscar had his vitamin and soft beef Milkbones after his Gravizon supplement and two Only Natural GI

Support capsules. He loves the soft beef Milkbones cookies, too! At 10:45 a.m., he drank some Ensure with two Slippery Elm capsules. Feeling encouraged, I made some ground veal with brown rice for him, and he ate ⅓ lb! At 5:15 p.m.., he ate another ⅓ lb of veal with brown rice. I gave him his Gravizon and red clover capsules accompanied by four to six medium-sized bone marrow cookies. He begged for more cookies at 6:30 p.m. and happily ate 10 more. Oscar was extremely weak, and tonight, Richard carried him upstairs.

March 13th: Oscar's weakened condition continued nearly all day long. Then, at 8 p.m., Richard gently lifted his body up to carry him upstairs, but once there he went off on his own! He's walking again!

March 14th: I greeted Oscar with a new little song this morning: "Superstar, here you are!" He perked up and looked at me with that familiar look as if to say, "What game are we going to play today?" Silly dog, Oscar! It was a rainy, somber day, but at least the snow is melting. I kept singing the phrase to him all day long, and will do so until the end. This dog keeps on rejuvenating himself…In the morning, he had ½ bottle of Ensure with his Gravizon capsule. At noon, he was able to eat a few ground veal meatballs and about eight bone marrow cookies. At 6 p.m., he had half a bottle of Ensure plus supplements, and by 8:30 p.m., he seemed hungry for more. "Superstar, here you are!" He ate half a large Milkbones cookie along with half of a big dog bowl of ground veal (big pieces) with Italian bread and his Gravizon and 2 Cellular Forte Max3 supplements.

March 15th: "Superstar, here you are!" At 8:30 a.m., Oscar gobbled up a large dog food bowl of French toast along with his Gravizon and Only Natural GI Support supplements.

At 2 p.m., he drank a full can of Ensure from his medium-sized heart bowl plus another Gravizon capsule and two red clover capsules. Dinner was similar to yesterday.

March 16th: At 8:30 a.m., Oscar ate French toast plus his Gravizon and Only Natural GI Support supplements. At 2 p.m., Richard surprised Oscar with a plain double hamburger that was served *Richard's style* in their usual hideout. Somehow, Richard was able to get in another Gravizon capsule during their time together, too. At 6 p.m., Oscar ate half of a big bowl of Italian bread and chicken mixture plus two more supplements.

March 17th: Around 9 a.m., Oscar had approximately eight pieces of an asiago bagel with a Gravizon capsule and one Cellular Forte Max3. At noon, he hungrily ate ⅔ of a large bowl of Italian bread and lamb mixture. Thankfully, he was hungry again in the evening, and ate ¾ of a bowl or more of the same lamb and bread mixture.

March 18th: This is the second consecutive week that Oscar has experienced some difficulty in going upstairs for the evening. Richard gladly carried him up the stairs, but Oscar was able to walk on his own from there. With the change in weather and the snow now melted, Oscar is still able to walk around on his own outside…Oscar's morning began with 10 Pedigree bone marrow cookies as he took his Gravizon and Only Natural GI Support supplements. At noon, Richard brought him a plain Chick-fil-A sandwich, and he was able to eat it all. I have a hunch that one of the workers here today gave Oscar a snack late in the afternoon — he didn't appear to be interested in eating until later on this evening. Then, he ate some Italian bread and chicken mixture.

March 19th: A better eating pattern continues. Oscar was up earlier today, and at 7 a.m., he had 10 bone marrow cookies with his Gravizon capsule and two Only Natural GI Support supplements. At 9:45 a.m., he had some vanilla Ensure in his heart bowl with two red clover capsules. By 2 p.m., he was happy to eat nearly ¾ of a plain Chick-fil-A sandwich. Later on, he ate pieces of roast chicken with his supplements. "Superstar, here you are!" At bedtime, Oscar had a minimum of a dozen bone marrow cookies and soft beef Milkbones cookies with his remaining supplements.

March 20th: Interestingly, Oscar ate his vitamin today along with the bone marrow cookie left in his sleeping spot as a little surprise. He later drank an entire bottle of vanilla Ensure from his medium-sized heart bowl followed by two supplements and a couple of bone marrow cookies. At noon, he had just a couple of pieces of a fresh hamburger, and at dinner he was able to eat a plain Chick-fil-A sandwich served *Richard's style*...After dinner, we took a ¾ mile walk. Oscar was slow and steady, and seemed glad to be walking with the wind on his face. He was happy to see the neighbors! Later on, Oscar climbed up the stairs to our bedroom by himself, and only once did he need a slight amount of help!

We readily welcome the new season, and embrace the hope that spring brings.

CHAPTER FOUR

This Spring With Oscar

❧ *Watching the Remedies Work*

March 21st: With the improvement in weather it seemed only right to infuse Oscar with new creative energy. "Superstar, here you are!" is a common melody in our household these days, and I might add that Winston and Richard also enjoy having the melody sung in reference to them!

I begin to hope and wish for Oscar to have the experience of discovering the reappearance of the Slippery Elm leaves on the backyard patch of young trees. We are not in charge of the end of this story, but it would be so wonderful to watch his expression of joy. As we are having a slow start to spring, the likelihood of this happening is less than certain.

Oscar's morning feeding pattern was the same today as yesterday. Around noon, I gave him a whole mashed sweet potato, which he thoroughly enjoyed, as well as nine bone marrow cookies. I give the cookies one at a time following each supplement. At 6:30 p.m., Oscar ate ¾ of a Chick-fil-A, plus his Only Natural GI Support and Gravizon supplements. Then, we noticed his interest in our dinner of BBQ pork roast baked with green peppers, onions, carrots, and pineapple. The BBQ sauce was a combination of 1 c. Heinz ketchup, 3 T. brown sugar, ¼ tsp. garlic powder, and two tsp. Worcestershire sauce. He was responding to the aroma! I decided to mix together some pork roast and rice and sauce in a bowl for him. *He had us in smiles in no time! Oscar devoured the bowl of pork with rice with some sauce. Appealing to his sweet tooth was an effective strategy to build his appetite!*

March 22nd: Oscar very happily ate his vitamin and cookie at 8 a.m. this morning. By 8:30 a.m., he appeared to be ready to eat, and ate five to seven pieces of cut-up French toast. At 4 p.m., Richard brought him a plain Chick-fil-A and Oscar ate it all. Later that evening, he had half of a bowlful of the BBQ pork roast with rice mixture. At bedtime, he had eight soft beef Milkbones cookies with his supplements and two bone marrow cookies.

March 23rd: Today is Easter Sunday. At 6:30 a.m., Oscar had his vitamin and a bone marrow cookie. Richard's breakfast today included some challah bread and both dogs enjoyed it very much! Oscar's appetite continues to be strong: at 10:30 a.m., he had half of a big bowl of cut-up French toast pieces with his Only Natural GI Support capsules. At 2 p.m. Oscar had a medium bowl of vanilla Ensure with his red clover supplements. Later this evening, he eagerly ate his favorite orange chicken with rice. At bedtime, he had 10 bone marrow cookies with his remaining supplements.

March 24th: Today began with a new twist! Oscar ate only his cookie at 7 a.m. and not his vitamin. Was this an act of silliness, or was this going to be a poor eating day? The answer soon became clear to us. At 9:15 a.m., Oscar took all of his supplements with eight bone marrow cookies. Around 12:30 p.m., he had half a can of vanilla Ensure in his heart bowl plus his Gravizon capsules. At 4:30 p.m., Oscar had a big bowl filled with orange chicken with rice.

March 25th: At 6:30 a.m., Oscar had his cookie and his vitamin, and by 8 a.m. he had his Gravizon capsules and Only Natural GI Support with bone marrow cookies. At 11 a.m., he happily ate mashed sweet potatoes with his red clover supplements. His appetite continued to be good throughout the day! Around 2 p.m., he was able to eat a whole plain Chick-fil-A sandwich. At 5:30 p.m., he seemed to be responding to the smells in the kitchen, so I offered him a bowlful of mashed potatoes with French chicken (brush the chicken with mustard, top with dry bread crumbs as well as dried basil, tarragon and chervil; pour melted butter over the chicken and then roast for an hour). He devoured nearly the entire bowl in no time! Between bites I was able to give him two red clover capsules plus his Gravizon supplement. At 9:30 p.m., he had numerous bone marrow cookies and soft beef Milkbones with all of his remaining supplements. *What happened next is very interesting—Oscar climbed upstairs to our bedroom on his own, and without any encouragement!* Could the remedies be restoring his body? **It's been nearly one month since he has been receiving the effective combination of remedies!**

March 26th: This was another excellent day. At 7 a.m., Oscar had his vitamin and bone marrow cookie, and by 8 a.m. he had bone marrow cookies along with his Gravizon and Only Natural GI Support supplements. At 11 a.m., he had a nice portion of mashed sweet potatoes with two red clover capsules. Around 1:30 p.m., he had a whole, plain Chick-fil-A sandwich, and ate it without any difficulty. At 5:30 p.m., Oscar had half a bowl of French chicken, mashed potatoes and Italian bread pieces mixed together along with Gravizon and two Cellular Forte Max3 tablets. *This was the second evening that Oscar walked upstairs with Winston without any assistance!*

March 27th: Today began much the same as the last two days. At 8 a.m., Oscar was resting on his soft bed of blankets and towels in the third garage as he waited for me to begin our morning routine. When I walked into the garage with their dog bowls, he got up and approached Winston's bowl and began to sniff it. His mischievous personality is back! He began to eat Winston's low-calorie dog food with his tail wagging, and thankfully, Winston was not in view. He also ate several bone marrow cookies along with one Gravizon capsule, two Only Natural GI Support capsules and one red clover supplement.

March 28th: My details on yesterday's eating were minimal due to the critical situation that arose regarding my Dad's health and treatment issues...Today began similarly to the pattern established this week. At 7 a.m., Oscar ate his vitamin and bone marrow cookie, and by 9 a.m. he was eager for more food. I gave him some warmed, mashed sweet potatoes (yams) and a Gravizon capsule, two red clover capsules and two Only Natural GI Support supplements. At noon, he ate a whole plain Chick-fil-A sandwich, and at 6:10 p.m. he had a bowl of BBQ pork roast and rice mixture. I drizzled more sauce on the mixture. In between his mouthfuls of food, I was able to give him one Gravizon capsule, two red clover capsules and two Only Natural GI Support supplements. He absolutely loves this meal! At 9:15 p.m., he finished his bowl of BBQ pork and rice. Finally, at 9:45 p.m., he had eight bone marrow cookies with a Gravizon capsule and two Cellular Forte Max3 tablets. This was a very good day!

March 29th: This was another very good day! Oscar ate his vitamin and cookie at 8 a.m., and some cut-up pieces of French toast around 9:30 a.m. At 12:30 p.m., he gobbled down a plain Chick-fil-A sandwich, and by 4:45 p.m., he ate nearly two cups of dry dog food. Happily, we took a 1⅓ mile walk, and Oscar did well! At 11 p.m., Oscar drank some Ensure with his supplements.

March 30th: At 9 a.m., Oscar had his vitamin and cookie, but refused any food offered to him until noon. Could the walk last night have affected him? At noon, I made a fresh yam for him and mashed it up nicely. It worked! He ate it enthusiastically! At 2 p.m., he ate ¾ of a plain quarter pound hamburger, and by 5 p.m., he ate half of a bowl of BBQ pork roast and rice. At 8 p.m., he ate the remainder of the bowl (minus a spoonful for Winston) with most of his supplements. Around 9:15 p.m., Oscar had about seven King Louis peanut butter cookies with the Cellular Forte Max3 tablets.

March 31st: The current medicine and cancer-reducing remedies appear to be working very well together! *One of our main goals was to help Oscar be able to eat healthy foods, and right now it appears that has been achieved. There is a rhythm to Oscar's eating pattern now...*At 6:30 a.m. today, Oscar had his vitamin and bone marrow cookie. At 8:45 a.m., he had a mashed yam, and at 11:15 a.m., he seemed eager to eat so I fed him a plain Chick-fil-A sandwich that he ate eagerly. At 4:30 p.m., he had ¾ of a quarter pound hamburger; at 8 p.m., he ate half a bowl of baked chicken and Italian bread mixture; and at bedtime he had six King Louis cookies with his supplements.

April 1st: Once again, at 6:30 a.m., Oscar had his vitamin and bone marrow cookie. At 7:50 a.m., he had mashed yams with two Only Natural GI Support capsules, his Gravizon supplements and two bone marrow cookies. At 1:30 p.m., Oscar ate ⅔ of a Chick-fil-A sandwich quite eagerly, but he refused an assortment of food offered to him at the evening mealtime. At 8 p.m., he was responsive to mashed yams with thin pieces of steak, and he ate half of the bowl. At 9:15 p.m., he ate King Louis cookies with the remaining five supplements.

April 2nd: Oscar's day began happily with his vitamin and bone marrow cookie. At 8:30 a.m., he ate a mashed yam, and at 10 a.m. he watched me leave to take Winston to his bath and grooming appointment. The look on Oscar's face indicated full awareness and acceptance. I didn't want to burden either dog with my sadness as it might affect Oscar's mood, so I emoted a tender cheerfulness as I presented him, with great ceremony, two large Milkbones cookies. A quick nuzzle of his strong face, and then we were off! Apparently, he ate them while we were away. At 12:30 p.m., Oscar ate ¾ of a plain Chick-fil-A sandwich. He didn't indicate any further interest in eating in the afternoon, and he rested the entire time. I gave him four bone marrow cookies with two red clover capsules as he lay peacefully in the family room. Thankfully, he clearly has no pain. At 9 p.m., he had a medium heart bowlful of Ensure plus two Cellular Forte Max3 tablets.

April 3rd: Today was a very good day! At 6:30 a.m., Oscar had his vitamin and bone marrow cookie, and at 8:30 a.m., he had a mashed yam with his morning supplements. He had a bone marrow cookie and some peanut butter pretzels from workers who were taking care of some repairs today. He still enjoys the attention! Around noon, he ate an entire plain Chick-fil-A sandwich. At 5 p.m., he was eager to eat, and I gave him some lean ground veal with cut-up pieces of his favorite Italian bread. At 8 p.m., he ate another portion of the same mixture. At 9 p.m., he walked over to the cookie cupboard, and I handed him two large Milkbones —Winston walked in the room at that very moment—I quickly turned it into a game of Milkbones. At 9:30 p.m., he had 3-4 King Louis peanut butter cookies with his remaining supplements for the day.

Time is running out for us. Will Oscar have another chance to experience the leaves?

✒ Smelling the Newly Budded Tree

April 4th: Oscar was so sad today. He ate his vitamin and cookie at 7 a.m., and also had his Chick-fil-A at noon. However, he seemed so sad. He is so very thin. The physical toll from his illness is obvious. Richard and I match our energy level with his these days, and as he is listless, our movements around him are consciously orchestrated with an extra dose of gentleness. I sat beside him quietly and nuzzled him as I sang softly,

"Superstar! Here you are!" These moments grip me deeply to my core, and I fight hard to manage my sorrow. Oscar's journey has been a gift to us, and his strength and courage will always be remembered. *He has provided us with a stellar example of how to live.*

Each time I walked past him today, I patted his sweet face and told him to "just rest." Winston—observer of all that is going on—appears to be more and more forlorn. If only he could talk! We tried to cheer Oscar with our usual games, but nothing worked until I put on my jacket and outdoor shoes, and instantly Oscar (and Winston) perked up. Obviously, we wouldn't be able to do a walk, but how about having some fun in the perennial garden? The rain had stopped, and while it was a bit foggy the temperature was in the low 50's. Oscar loved being outdoors, and I hoped this would cheer him. I went out through the garage, gathered my pruning shears and a garbage can, and then looked behind me. Two beautiful dogs were in tow! They loved the activity and the surprise! Tails began to wag, and, seeing this, I felt so much better, and I began to focus on pruning the butterfly bush. Soon, two happy dogs were hunting around the gardens as they kept careful watch on me. I soaked in the joy of the moment as the three of us shared some quiet fun outside. This was such a beautiful way to end the day!

April 5th: During the night, I heard Oscar eating a bone marrow cookie that I had placed beside him on his therapeutic bed upstairs. I smiled in hearing the noise, and could only imagine what Winston was thinking at this very moment! Maybe Winston was glad to hear the noise, too. This morning, Oscar ate his cookie and vitamin at 8 a.m. Mid-morning, he ate half a bowlful of French toast, and I decided not to interrupt his eating to give him a Gravizon capsule. He is acting so weak and depressed; after he ate his Chick-fil-A sandwich he seemed somewhat stronger, so I decided to take a short, slow walk down the street with them. Various neighbors called out to us or came over to say hello, and Oscar's face became noticeably happier. However, I also noticed that his balance was off, so I didn't allow him to stand still for long, concerned that we might not be able to make it home. His paws are so lean that they resemble webbed feet. However, slow and steady, Oscar walked the ¾ mile loop, and took his time enjoying the sunshine and sniffing the branches of the trees and the smells in the open patch of field along the side of the road. *As I observed Oscar, it occurred to me that this very well may be his last walk.* Poor Winston. He wanted to walk briskly, but I needed to hold him back again and again.

While out to dinner at Crave restaurant that evening, we mentioned Oscar's situation to our waitress. It was obvious she was an animal lover. She listened carefully, and then resumed her other responsibilities. Moments later, she appeared with a doggy bag for Oscar! Inside the bag was a gift from the chef: a beautiful Oso Buco bone! We were deeply touched by their kindness and couldn't wait to show the beautiful big bone to Oscar. When we returned home, I pulled Winston aside, and Richard and Oscar went into their little hideout in the third garage. Sadly, he appeared disinterested and was unable to react to it...Later on, we noticed that he was dragging his front paw, and Richard immediately picked him up and carried him upstairs to rest on his bed. Winston stood there taking it all in. Once upstairs, Winston came over to Oscar's bed to have some treats while Oscar had his cookies and supplements. I was amazed that Oscar looked at me to give him his supplements — he continues to surprise us!

April 6th: We heard Oscar walking around during the night, and once again, he discovered the bone marrow cookie I had hidden beside his bed. It was wonderful to hear his happy crunching! At 8 a.m., Oscar ate his vitamin and cookie...*His diarrhea has returned...I now interpret these bouts as the completion of a cycle, and feel that the diarrhea releases the toxins...* At 11 a.m., Oscar ate nearly all of a plain quarter pound hamburger, and at 3:30 p.m. he ate nearly all of a plain double hamburger served *Richard's-style*. At 3:45 p.m., he ate six carob sandwich cookies that were filled with peanut butter. He is having a very wobbly day, and we feel our time left with him is short. All morning long, I kept thinking of other ways that I could cheer him, and then in the late afternoon I came up with an idea.

I made a spontaneous decision to head outside to work in the perennial garden. When I walked through the garage, Oscar was resting peacefully on his soft blankets, and Winston was lying outside on the grass. As always, the side door of the garage was open for the dogs to have easy access to their food and water bowls and also their soft resting area. I cuddled their faces as I passed them, and then proceeded to walk toward the gated area where Oscar had discovered the slippery elm patch. There was a foggy mist all day long, and the sky was dark and gloomy overhead. Because of the rather cold temperatures spring arrived slowly this year, and we were longing to see buds on the trees. I wanted to check on the slippery elm patch, so I opened the latched gate. What happened next is etched in my memory forever...

Hearing the noise of the gate opening, a very wobbly Oscar got up from his resting area and came out of the garage to see what I was up to. I watched him as he slowly, carefully walked toward me, and I stepped back so that he could enter the gated area before I did. He immediately went over to the branches of the young trees, and using his nose, swept up the branch as far as he could reach. Much to my delight, on the frail slippery elm branches were buds of leaves for the new growing season. Oscar licked his lips, and his tail began to wag happily as he proceeded to sniff the entire patch of branches.

At this moment I needed to make a quick decision: do I head inside to get the camera to capture this moment on film, or would it be better for me to remain here with Oscar to savor this beautiful moment? I chose the latter. Then, as if he knew what I had been contemplating and agreed with my choice, he turned to look at me, his tail wagging with great happiness, and I hugged him as he happily remembered the leaves.

The leaves are coming back, Oscar!

↬ Love always, Oscar

April 7th: Today, I promised myself that, if possible, Oscar would once again have a chance to enjoy all of his favorite foods and cookies. At 6:30 a.m., he had his bone marrow cookie plus his vitamin. His face was so very sad and I believe he is grieving. He knows what we know. He wanted to walk down the stairs without our help, but when he fell, Richard was there to catch him and carried him all the remaining way down. Once downstairs, he was able to walk on his own. He didn't want any sweet potatoes, or anything else for that matter, when I checked on him mid-morning, but around 11:30 a.m., I heard his quiet yelping barks in delight as he heard Richard's car come into the main garage. He was already out in the third garage resting on his soft blankets where he and Richard always had their secret feedings, so he may have been barking with excitement as a surprise was about to be delivered! Amazingly, he ate the entire plain Chick-fil-A sandwich. Later on, he had two bites of hamburger along with six carob sandwich cookies filled with peanut butter, and one Gravizon capsule along with two Only Natural Pet GI Support capsules. A later feeding consisted of a small amount of orange chicken with rice.

April 8th: At 6:40 a.m., Oscar had his vitamin and bone marrow cookie. At 8:30 a.m., I brought out the small heart bowl and filled it with vanilla Ensure. He wouldn't drink on his own at first, but when I put my finger in the bowl and showed it to him, he drank some and then sighed deeply. At 11:30 a.m. he ate nearly ¾ of a plain Chick-fil-A. His evening feeding consisted of a large bowl filled with orange chicken and rice, and he ate steadily without interruption. Cookies and supplements were given as usual at bedtime.

April 9th: Oscar had his vitamin and bone marrow cookie at 7 a.m., and then proceeded to walk down the stairs by himself. We were right there beside him and walked at his pace. Winston had already scampered down the steps and was waiting there for us at the bottom of the stairs, watching Oscar very carefully. At 8:30 a.m., Oscar ate a chunk of canned tuna in water along with two pieces of an asiago bagel. At noon, Oscar ate all of the remaining orange chicken and rice! His evening feeding consisted of half of a double hamburger. At 9:30 p.m., he had eight carob sandwich cookies filled with peanut butter along with all of his supplements.

April 10th: At 7:15 a.m., Oscar ate his vitamin and bone marrow cookie upstairs. I found it interesting that when I petted him, he wanted to lick off my hand cream! Just like old times! He came downstairs independently, but slipped on the descending step in the kitchen as he was entering the family room. He was able to steady himself, and his fierce pride enabled him to walk out to the backyard. At 8:30 a.m., Oscar ate 20 small flavored Milkbones, two pieces of hamburger and four beef-flavored pill pockets (four supplements tucked inside). The large tumor under his tongue has shrunk in size and is almost invisible now! His tongue is now a brighter shade of pink than the sides of his mouth! At 3:45 p.m., he ate an entire plain Chick-fil-A sandwich. He was wobbly this afternoon — the weather was in the low 50's and while the day began gloomy, it turned into a sunny day. His evening feeding consisted of BBQ pork roast with rice, and he ate a large bowlful without any difficulty. It is wonderful knowing that he is able to eat again, and that there are no more growling noises from his stomach.

April 11th: At 6:30 a.m., Oscar had his vitamin and bone marrow cookie, and at 8:30 a.m., he took all of his supplements with peanut butter pretzels and about 20 bone marrow cookies. He doesn't seem to be interested in mashed yams anymore. The weather was very gloomy today, but we know that sunny days will soon be here! At noon, Oscar ate nearly the entire (large) bowl of BBQ pork roast with rice. He rested most of the day with an occasional walk outside to experience the breeze. At 7 p.m., he ate another large bowl of BBQ pork roast with rice. Richard carried him upstairs to his bed, with Winston walking up right behind them.

April 12th: Oscar appeared to be very weak and disinterested in food this morning, so I did not bring an assortment of things over to him to encourage his eating. Instead, I placed several bone marrow cookies and some small, flavored Milkbones beside him should he become interested in eating them…The morning was extremely stressful as Richard and I needed to be elsewhere, and I wished I could remain at home. It seemed as if Oscar was beginning to slip away from us. I felt conflicted about leaving, but the commitment was a critical one. Winston was good company for Oscar in the garage while we were away…Upon our return home, Oscar was more alert and somewhat better, and he was able to eat another large bowl of BBQ pork roast with rice.

April 13th: Oscar was very weak and listless this morning, and Richard carried him downstairs. The time has come for us to call Dr. Heller to discuss euthanization. When I returned home later that morning, Oscar appeared alert and had energy, and he was able to eat half of a double hamburger. However, I later watched him get up, walk 20 steps and then tumble. He is so thin that even I am able to carry him now. Our brave and beloved Oscar, the time is nearing when we will need to say our loving good-bye. Bravo, Special One! Your work was done with valor! Winston appears very stressed with the developments, and we tried to comfort him and Oscar while they rested together on the soft blankets in the third garage…Later on, Oscar was able to eat another large bowl of BBQ pork with rice and appeared to be walking well and without hesitation. Was it time to euthanize him, or not? At bedtime, he looked at me to give him his cookies and supplements — I gave him a Gravizon capsule and two of the Cellular Forte Max3 capsules.

April 14th: Sadly, our last day with our precious Oscar has arrived. At 6:30 a.m., Oscar ate his vitamin and bone marrow cookie. Richard carried him all the way downstairs and into the family room this morning, and we were soon able to see that Oscar was incapable of walking more than a few steps. We carried him outdoors and brought him back to his favorite spot these days—the soft blanket area beside their feeding bowls. Richard put in a call to Dr. Heller's office and learned that his day was completely filled with surgeries, some due to emergencies and others for some very sick dogs...We had formulated a back-up plan in the event that Dr. Heller was unavailable. Dr. Ben Pearson had been recommended to us, as we were interested in euthanizing Oscar in a manner reflecting the greatest kindness and gentleness. While we waited for a returned phone call from Dr. Pearson, I kept close watch on Oscar, making certain to check on him every few minutes. This time, when I opened the door to enter the garage, Winston came rushing over to me with a frantic expression on his face! Oscar had fallen in the garage as he was trying to go outside to relieve himself. I picked Oscar up and carried him outside, but he couldn't stand on his own very long...when he was once again back on the soft towels and blankets where he was comfortable, warm and safe, I cleaned up his "accident" as he watched me. I maintained a cheery sound to my voice, and then went inside to report the latest development to Richard, and to see if he had been able to make contact with Dr. Pearson. They were actually conversing when I entered the room, so I decided to go back to check on the dogs. Once again, Winston came rushing over to me as I opened the door to the garage, and I quickly understood why. Oscar had fallen again and his facial expression was one of humiliation from having a second accident. I gently lifted him up, and carefully cleaned him. Emotionally, this was my moment of knowing that euthanization was, indeed, the humane thing to do. I laid him down on fresh and even softer towels and blankets. He was shaking all over, and his eyes were imploring me to help! I covered him everywhere except for his face, and I sat there, facing him, and looked into his eyes. Not much longer, beloved Oscar! Once again, I thanked him for his goodness, and for the gift of being our dog. I told him what he meant to me and to everyone who knew him. The time had come, and we were both at peace.

It was a very quiet ride to Dr. Pearson's office, and Richard and I kept turning around to check on Oscar. He had no expression on his face, but his eyes were aware of all that was happening. He was resting comfortably in his bed that was in the rear of the car, and we had positioned his head against the bumper pad for support. Once we arrived at Dr. Pearson's office, I stayed with Oscar and Richard. Much to my surprise, Dr. Pearson came outside to the car to meet Oscar. His respect and love for animals was clearly apparent, and his gentleness with Oscar was deeply touching. He wanted to help carry Oscar inside, and so I walked behind Richard and Dr. Pearson, taking in the view of his office building and the wooded areas surrounding it. I liked the appliquéd Statue of Liberty sketches on the side window, and I also liked the wholesome feeling once I was inside.

Oscar, Richard and I, along with Dr. Pearson, shared the next hour together as we honored, with dignity, this remarkable dog's life. Dr.

Pearson asked about his illness and was genuinely interested in the remedies we utilized. We shared our feelings about this long healing journey, and also our concerns about Winston and his issues of loss. Dr. Pearson spoke ever so kindly about just loving Winston. We also talked about some things that might help Winston with this transition. Richard asked Dr. Pearson to send one of the growths on Oscar's body to the lab for analysis, so that we might learn more about his cancer.

Oscar's journey ended with both of us and a compassionate vet who honored his meaning in our lives. Oscar's healing journey and slow good-bye was one of the most loving experiences in our lifetime. He taught us how to live. Now, it was up to us to share what we learned.

If we grow in love, we may expect to Love, always.

CHAPTER FIVE:

Epilogue

❧ *Winston's Response*

On the way home from Dr. Pearson's office, I prepared myself for the necessary task of conveying to Winston that Oscar would not be coming home. When we pulled into our driveway, Winston was waiting for us at the front window. As we pulled into the garage my idea came together. I reached for Oscar's blue blanket as I stepped out of the car, and walked over to the house entrance. I opened the door and Winston came running out, looking at me for a response. I slowly knelt in front of him and showed him Oscar's blanket. He paused and stared at it, and then put his nose deep into the folds of the blanket to sniff it. I spoke softly saying, "I am so terribly sorry, Winston." In our silence, it seemed as if he was piecing it all together. All of a sudden, he uttered a noise similar to a "hmm." With that, he seemed to understand the finality of the fact. He walked on past us and out into the backyard.

That evening, I cleaned their entire eating area as well as the dogs' resting area in the third garage, and put a new set of bowls out for Winston where both sets had previously been. Winston watched everything I did that night. The next day, I bought a new leash and brand new treats as well. He and I took our first walk without Oscar, and Winston weaved from the left to the right as if he were attempting to fill the void. In time, he was able to walk straight again, but he quickly became incapable of walking more than 1⅓ miles at a time. Each walk ended with a long pause in front of the very old and magnificent Slippery Elm tree in our front yard. He paused and sat there as if in tribute to their times of enjoying the leaves there together. Although he did eat the leaves from the seedlings in the gated area in the backyard, he never again ate a leaf from the magnificent Slippery Elm tree in our front yard.

For 14 months, Winston's mood was affected by the loss, and even though we did many new and different things, he only seemed to want to lie there in the family room. We walked in the village, I baked him cookies, provided him with plenty of Chew Lotta's (which he licked—this activity became his favorite pastime), and I tried to take him on regular trips to the park. We created new associations and brought him to the Perfect Pet grooming team who were delighted to take care of him. But, his somberness did not ease, and we were reluctant to travel as we thought he might not be able to survive the separation.

However, the last seven months of his life were different. He reinvented himself thanks to the kindness of an extraordinary dog lover named Anne Weiser. One day, I came across a business card for the Orrville Pet Spa & Resort in Wooster, Ohio that someone had given me years earlier. The woman had mentioned the custom care offered there, and I decided to drive over to see Orrville for myself. The facility and staff did not disappoint me! Their dog "suites" were complete with low beds, and some even had gated views of the front desk. Freshly baked cookies were given to each dog daily, there were play periods with the staff, and they even made arrangements for gentle play dates for senior dogs like Winston. There was a TV in each suite that aired the channel, "Animal Planet." While traveling, dog owners could log online to view how their pet was doing. Anne and her entire staff were compassionate and sensitive to the recent events in Winston's life, and they seemed to be very interested in loving him.

We proceeded slowly in exposing Winston to the staff and the facility, and gave him short little field trips over to the pet resort. He found the displays of stuffed animals and squeaky toys on low cots in the reception area to be very "cool." He checked these out every time he visited as the staff made a point of rearranging them! He also liked the cat area that was off to the right. He was tall enough to see through the window and appeared to be just fascinated in watching what they were doing! Initially, "Mr. Winston" was given the job of being a dog counselor, and he was allowed to visit the very sad Golden Retrievers who were missing their owners. Anne brought him into her office as her heart was pulling for him. Winston was fussed over by the sweetest and cutest 16-year-old girls one could ever hope to meet, and in short, the unique blend of love and fascination brought him back to life. Once again, he enjoyed being with people and other animals, and his tail wagged a lot.

Winston passed away at home 21 months after Oscar died. Moments prior to his passing, Richard and I said our goodbyes to him, and he lay there in the family room close beside me. His legs had already lost their ability to move, and we knew that death was near. Because of his need to be dominant all of these years, Winston hadn't always wanted or needed to be hugged (which was so different from Oscar), so at this moment we gave him plenty of space. But, when he began to make all sorts of noises, I got up to sit beside him. He put his head deep into my arms and sighed. He wanted to be hugged! He did that one more time. Then, he pulled his head back and turned on his side, his legs extended out in front of him. His eyes began to look as if they were focused on something far in the distance. Suddenly, Winston began to make happy barking sounds and his legs began to move as if he were galloping! His front and back legs were in perfect sync. He was running, and running so fast, and barking with absolute joy!!!

And then, the whirring sound of blowing air filled the room. Air began to flow out of Winston and it moved the long hairs near his tail. It was at this moment that life progressively began to leave his body. Ever so slowly, his tail stopped wagging, his rear legs returned to their previous stiff position, his stomach no longer moved up and down, his front legs stopped all motion, and then finally, his head lay still. His beautiful passing was a gift to be shared. We believe that Winston and Oscar were reunited, and are now playing together again.

⁕ Dr. Heller's Response

Richard and I gratefully acknowledge the genuine caring and kindness that was shown to Oscar and Winston by Dr. Heller and his fine staff. I wish to offer special recognition and my profound gratitude to Joyce Carrick, whose support for Oscar's journey was unlike anyone else's at the time. A short time after Oscar's passing, Dr. Heller sent us the following note:

"I'm very sorry about your loss of Oscar. I did not think that he would be here eleven months from the time of his diagnosis. The day you called I was backlogged with appointments and could not get away. Someday, I hope to read your book about Oscar's journey."

❧ Dr. Pearson's Response

Richard and I anxiously awaited the lab results on the exposed growth from Oscar's body that Dr. Pearson had sent to be tested. When the test results were available, we met with him to learn the answer. Interestingly, the results indicated an absence of malignancy.

Could it be that the combination of remedies were working at the time he passed away?

Dr. Pearson and his staff provided us with tremendous support and encouragement on this project and were extremely compassionate regarding Winston's needs until he passed away. We will be forever grateful that Dr. Pearson opened his heart to us on this journey.

❧ Leaving a Legacy

The buds on the Slippery Elm trees that Oscar had the opportunity to smell, just days before he passed away, opened shortly thereafter. It was gratifying to watch the patch of seedlings grow by leaps and bounds during that spring and summer. They were young trees by now, and the more they grew, the more they became intertwined with each other. I began to wonder if it was possible to transplant them to other locations so they could have a chance to thrive. As the United Plant Savers Association has placed the Slippery Elm tree on the endangered species list, it seemed that working to reverse the situation would be a way to honor Oscar's legacy. Richard and I were enthused about the possibility of doing this.

During the fall, our tree doctor, Mr. Frank Wilcox, determined that two, possibly three, might be able to survive such a move, but he was tentative about predicting the likelihood of success. We decided to proceed with the project anyway. On a beautiful fall day, Mr. Wilcox carefully and artfully removed the three strongest trees from the cluster. Each was a different size. We decided to plant the medium-sized tree near some pine trees in our front yard. The smallest tree was planted fairly close to the magnificent Slippery Elm tree alongside the road. However, the tallest and most perfectly formed tree was offered as a gift to my beloved friends, Congressman Ralph Regula and Dr. Mary Regula. Their love of trees has been life long, and the significance of gifting them with a giving tree seemed analogous to our treasured friendship.

When I called them to see if they would be interested in having the tree, their excitement grew as they talked back and forth with each other. A gifted and accomplished gardener, Mary knew all the right questions to ask so they would be able to select a good location for the young tree. The placement they chose was very close to the entrance of their family farm, right beside the horse coral. I was able to capture the actual moment of planting on film. Both Mary and Congressman Regula were present when Mr. Wilcox ceremoniously performed his task. Just as I imagined, the horses came over to share in the excitement of this special day of planting.

Today, this impressive tree grows stronger and taller with each passing year. It already has an awe-inspiring and commanding presence at the entrance to the Regula's farm, symbolic of its giving legacy. While the smallest of the young trees was unable to survive the transplant, the medium-sized tree in our front yard is growing beautifully. Shoots of young and healthy seedlings are sprouting at the base of the tree, and this would have made Oscar and Winston very happy.

Q & A WITH THE AUTHOR

Introduction to the Appendices

What are the Appendices?
Jan: This is a section of the book that is devoted to how-to-find Oscar's treatment remedies, and also to sharing information about how I came to discover them.

Why are you sharing this information?
Jan: I am hoping that the effective combination of remedies that were discovered will help other dogs live even longer than Oscar lived.

Is this part of Oscar's legacy?
Jan: Yes.

Are there other reasons for including the Appendices in the book?
Jan: It is my hope that more information will be learned about dog cancer through others' administration of the same remedies. It is my greatest hope that readers will want to pick-up where we left off! The effective combination of remedies that enabled Oscar to eat were,

unfortunately, discovered late in the course of his illness, but perhaps another dog might be helped if treatments are received sooner.

Do you have any other hopeful messages for the reader?
Jan: Just imagine! If other dog owners were to capture the adventurous spirit, additional treatments and remedies may be discovered as well.

Please join in the effort to make strides against dog cancer by reading the following information provided in the appendices.

Notes

Notes

Appendix I: Slippery Elm and the Original Essiac Formula

Several articles provided me with excellent information about Slippery Elm's effectiveness when combined with other herbs in treating cancer. This information became available to me thanks to the helpfulness of a wonderful new friend. I met Tammie Young, a Cherokee descendant, at a Native American Indian Veteran's Center (www.naivc1.com) event. She was a guest speaker for that evening's program, and spoke about "Natural Herbs and Their Usage," a topic she knew much about as the information had been given to her from her mother, who, in turn, had learned it from relatives of her generation. Traditionally, this information was passed down from one generation to another in order to preserve the rich Native American Indian heritage, and also to provide a means of additional income for one's family.

After Tammy finished her presentation, we had an opportunity to talk about her specific knowledge about Slippery Elm. In answering my questions, she mentioned that the original Essiac tea recipe was available on the internet. I was greatly surprised to hear this as I assumed it would be a protected trade secret! However, true to the spirit of Nurse Caisse's work and mission, this information is available online and is to be shared.

Listed below are some of the titles of the articles available at http://www.healthfreedom.info/cancerEssiac.htm:

"ESSIAC INFO." This Essiac information page is the navigation page to the www.healthfreedom.info Web site.

"I Was Canada's Cancer Nurse: The Story of ESSIAC," by Rene M. Caisse, R.N. This article provides a fascinating history of this remarkable woman, the events that led to her doctor-observed research, and the opening of her free cancer clinic. Because her treatment methods resulted in many cured patients, she was tormented for nearly five decades by a group of individuals even though she "was working with nine of the most eminent physicians in Toronto, and was giving (my) treatment only at their request." It was the direct evidence of her effective treatment, and the petition of 55,000 signatures (which included 387 patients and many doctors) that kept her from being imprisoned.

"Proof of the Authentic, Original Essiac Tea Formula: Mary McPherson's Affidavit." A copy of Exhibit A, Mary McPherson's sworn affidavit dated December 23, 1994 is provided in this article. Her handwritten description of the Essiac tea formula and recipe is actually provided here –"the only verifiable, legal evidence of Rene Caisse's Essiac formula."

"The Authentic, Original Essiac Tea Formula & Recipe." The formula and recipe according to the transcription of Mary McPherson's affidavit are printed out in this article.

"The Truth About Essiac: Rene Caisse and her Herbal Cancer Treatment, Essiac." This article provides some very interesting information about all of the herbs in the Essiac tea formula, including Slippery Elm "the only Essiac herb native to North America." I greatly appreciated learning, "Some people drink the Essiac dregs (particles that settle on the bottom), others don't. Some people give the Essiac dregs to their pets or farm animals as a health food. Many people have reported the same or similar health benefits with their pets that humans are reporting. The dregs can also be used topically as a poultice."

Notes

Appendix II: Only Natural Pet GI Support

The information contained in this appendix is about Only Natural Pet GI Support, the first remedy I used in Oscar's treatment. I discovered the product in the colorful Only Natural Pet Store catalog that miraculously arrived in our mail one day.

This product is a gastrointestinal supplement for cats and dogs. Among the ingredients selected for this quality product is Slippery Elm bark. When I read about this supplement and its ingredients, I immediately decided to use it for Oscar's care. According to www.onlynaturalpet.com, it is helpful for a dog or cat that has regular episodes of "vomiting, diarrhea, constipation, or indigestion." It "delivers advanced gastrointestinal support," and is comprised of "a unique combination of probiotics, vitamins, herbs, health-building co-factors and enzymes. This best-selling formula is ideal for animals suffering from chronic or recurrent poor digestion, food allergies, or irritable bowel issues." This product worked extremely well on Oscar's symptoms.

Ninety-six product reviews were written about Only Natural Pet GI Support at the time of this research, and the comments were categorized into pros, cons and best uses categories. All of the information listed about the product on the company's Web site may be helpful for a concerned dog owner. Please note that the Only Natural Pet Store reserves the right to change their Web site content at any time. They update the site content often, and were about to launch a new Web site at the time of this printing. Therefore, the same content may be laid out differently when the reader accesses the site.

～ Notes

꧁ Appendix III: Only Natural Pet Immune Strengthener

The Only Natural Pet Immune Strengthener is the second remedy I discovered in the Only Natural Pet Store catalog. According to the store's Web site, http://www.onlynaturalpet.com, "When your pet's health has been compromised by a serious problem or as a result of normal aging, our Immune Strengthener's blend of natural vitamins, herbs, antioxidants and mushrooms can provide immune system support to help your dog or cat fight chronic health issues while supporting organ function."

Further, "this formula supplies a wide range of antioxidant ingredients to foster the maximum reduction of free radical damage to cells. We also included some of the finest known immune-supportive herbal ingredients like Cat's Claw and Reishi, Shitake, and Maitake mushroms—three of the most effective and commonly used mushrooms in Chinese herbal medicine."

"One of the best selling and most popular items in our Only Natural Pet product line, Immune Strengthener consistently draws rave reviews on www.onlynaturalpet.com (One hundred two reviews were written at the time of this writing; their stories follow the product description.) General immune system stress, general cardiovascular dysfunctions, and general liver impairment and kidney conditions," are typical health issues that may respond to this product.

Again, it is necessary for me to mention that the Only Natural Pet Store reserves the right to change their Web site content at any time.

They update site content often, and were about to launch a new Web site at the time of this printing. Therefore, the same content may be laid out differently when the reader accesses the site.

Initially, this product worked very well for Oscar, but it was eliminated from his treatment plan when I determined the most effective grouping of remedies for his particular illness.

✏ Notes

Notes

Appendix IV: PhytoPharmica Cellular Forté with IP-6 & Inositol

The information within this appendix pertains to PhytoPharmica Cellullar Forté with IP-6 & Inositol, but this product is now listed as Integrative Therapeutics Cellular Forte with IP-6 & Inositol on the Only Natural Pet Store Web site. The product number remains the same (#106001), but the name of the item has changed.

According to the Only Natural Pet Store Web site: http://www.onlynaturalapet.com/product "Integrative Therapeutics Cellular Forté with Ip-6 and Inositol provides nutritional support of immune function including healthy cell development and natural killer cell activity. It boosts the natural cellular defenses by increasing levels of inositol phosphates in cells to help strengthen and enhance the immune system. IP-6 is found in the bran of brown rice and inositol, part of the vitamin B family, both help support the immune system."

This supplement performs in the following ways:

- Boosts the body's natural defenses

- Enhances healthy cell growth

- Dramatically increases natural killer cell activity

- No artificial flavoring, coloring or preservatives

- No corn, wheat, yeast or gluten

- No dairy products

- No salt, soy or sugar

- Ingredients of animal origin

Also posted on the product information page are paragraphs about healthy cell development and natural killer cells. This information was very interesting to me in light of Oscar's condition. Our grip on his illness was slipping, and we needed more of an underpinning to our treatment plan. Because of these reasons, I decided to order this product. It worked well, but in the end it was eliminated from the treatment plan due to the stronger properties of the other products.

~~ Notes

✒ Notes

Appendix V: NF Spectrum Probiotic

It was apparent that Oscar was greatly troubled by his intermittent problem with diarrhea. In fact, treating the problem of diarrhea is a cornerstone of the treatment plan for a beloved pet suffering with cancer. Why? Chronic diarrhea kept Oscar from wanting to be with us as he was never certain when he would need to dash out the "doggy-door." But what if there was no doggy door? He would have given us the indication that he needed to go outside immediately. Golden's do not like to create messes (it seemed as if he was ashamed of himself when he had an accident). Keeping a close connectedness with us made him come to life, and he was able to show his personality! Therefore, this was important to maintain his morale. I understand these things much better now, years after his illness. It is so important to eliminate this problem so your pet may feel more normal, and so that everyone can focus more on wellness.

I am excited to share that including probiotics in his treatment plan seemed to help eliminate this symptom. This is the fourth remedy I discovered from the Only Natural Pet Store. Their Web site, www.onlynaturalpet.com, lists the benefits of probiotics as listed below:

"• Essential for use during and after antibiotic treatment to replace "friendly" intestinal bacteria destroyed by antibiotics.

• Aid in digestion and suppress disease-causing bacteria.

• Aid in preventing and treating diarrhea.

- Combats the overgrowth of "unhealthy" organisms in the gastrointestinal tract (a condition that can cause diarrhea and may occur from antibiotic use).

- Alleviate symptoms of inflammatory bowel disease.

- Helps prevent and/or reduce the recurrence of yeast infections, urinary tract infections, and cystitis (bladder inflammation).

- Lactobacillus sporogenes binds cholesterol in the gut, and may inhibit the cholesterol-producing enzyme HMG CoA Reductase."

When Oscar's stool was normal, he seemed to be happier and more engaged with us. This was an extremely significant remedy. I am so thrilled that we were finally able to manage this symptom of dog cancer! This is a wonderful remedy to include in the treatment plan for dog cancer.

Notes

Notes

Appendix VI: ONPS B.S.S.T. Herbal Formula

According to http://www.onlynaturalpet.com, the Only Natural Pet B.S.S.T. Herbal Formula contains the four herbs in the famous Essiac formula, developed by the Canadian nurse, Rene Caisse. The herbs in the formula have a long history of use in herbal medicine traditions of many cultures. Limited research has been conducted with the Essiac formula and its individual herbal ingredients, and specific health-supportive properties of the herbs have been identified. These herbs may help maintain cellular health, purify the blood, and help eliminate destroyed tissues and toxic residues."

"Our B.S.S.T. Herbal Formula is designed to help strengthen the innate defense mechanisms of the body to support the immune system's ability to fight pathogenic and system-degenerative ailments and to destroy abnormal cells. Together, the herbs in the formula produce synergistic effects that enhance each herb's individual beneficial properties." Customer reviews are very positive regarding the results they have had with BSST.

"B.S.S.T. contains the following high quality herbs:

- Burdock Root

- Sheep's Sorel Leaf

- Slippery Elm Bark

- Turkey Rhubarb Root"

As this product was available in liquid form only, it needed to be added to Oscar's water. However, he detected the change and then refused to drink his water. I realized he was disinterested due to the change in the taste of his water. Oscar and Winston always loved to drink water! They were in the habit of drinking a large amount of water throughout the day due to the their high activity level. I did not add the drops to Oscar's food as it seemed he did not like the taste.

This product did not work for us despite the quality of the nutrients and the very positive customer reviews.

～ Notes

Notes

Appendix VII: Oscar's Favorite Orange Chicken Recipe

Ingredients:

1 whole roasting chicken (select a free range chicken, no hormones added or a vegetarian diet type)

1 box of Uncle Ben's Original Long Grain & Wild Rice Mix

1 can of orange segments, drained

1 can of sliced water chestnuts, drained

½ jar of Smucker's orange marmalade

¼ cup of Wishbone fat-free Italian Dressing

"Butter" flavored Pam natural vegetable oil spray (or your favorite brand)

Directions:

Pre-heat your oven to 400°. Rinse the chicken well with cold water, inside and out, and pat it completely dry with paper towels. Prepare a pan for roasting. Spray the pan with "butter" flavor Pam or another natural vegetable oil spray. Pour contents of the box of rice into a deep sauce pan, and pour in the contents of the seasonings package as well.

Pour 1¼ c. of water into the saucepan, and stir mixture slowly. Simmer or cook on low heat until much of the water has been absorbed into the rice (note: the rice will still be hard). Add the sliced water chestnuts and the orange segments to the rice mixture and stir carefully. Fill the cavity of the chicken with the rice mixture, and then place the chicken into the prepared roasting pan, surrounding the chicken with the remaining rice mixture. Next, put ½ jar of orange marmalade into a small bowl, and pour in ¼ cup of the Wishbone Italian dressing into the bowl and blend well. Baste the chicken with this marinade—spoon it over the chicken, making sure to drizzle some also over the rice. Make more of the marinade mixture, if necessary, as the entire chicken needs to be coated. Cover the rice surrounding the chicken with aluminum foil, but leave the chicken exposed so it will turn brown.

Cooking time is approximately 2 hours in a regular oven, or 1¼ hours in an oven with a convection bake mode. This is a delicious chicken recipe. I truly hope that you and your pet will enjoy the wonderful aroma and the very good flavor!

Notes

Notes

Appendix VIII: Gravizon

This appendix contains information about a product named Gravizon™. According to www.amazonbioenergetics.com/gravizon.htm, Gravizon™ "is an enhanced immune, circulatory and lymphatic formula containing the whole-leaf spagyric extract of the Graviola tree, a small evergreen tree from the Amazon. Rainforest natives have a rich history of using this herb for its profound healing properties—among them, immune, circulatory and lymphatic support. Research since the 1940's has validated and expanded understanding of this herb and its unique phyto-nutritional qualities. It is currently under intense study for its potential to possibly assist in blocking free radicals and abnormal cell growth."

"Gravizon™ blends Graviola with three powerful Amazon Herb formulas: Arcozon™, which maintains the body's defense system; Envirozon™, which helps cleanse the body of toxins; Recovazon™, which supports the body in healing itself. Gravizon™ also incudes Camu Camu, Sangre de Drago, and Abuta. This synergistic blend promotes exceptional immune function."

This product is extraordinary! We saw great results within a short amount of time! I am very excited to share this incredible product with all of you. It is available from www.amazonherbs.net. Click on "Quick Order" on the top right, then follow the instructions. I purchased it in pill form rather than in liquid form due to Oscar's personal preference.

Notes

Appendix IX: Red Clover

This appendix provides information about a very interesting herb by the name of red clover. After it was suggested to me, I researched it online and then purchased it from our local health food store. The bottle of red clover supplements (capsules) was on display among the many natural supplements on the shelves. The results were outstanding on reducing the growth under Oscar's tongue! This is a very powerful and fascinating herb to study.

According to the University of Maryland Medical Center's Web site http://www.umm.edu/altmed/articles/red-clover-000270), "Red clover is a wild plant that is used for grazing cattle and other animals. It has also been used medicinally to treat a number of conditions. Traditionally, these have included cancer, whooping cough, respiratory problems, and skin inflammations, such as psoriasis and eczema. Red clover was thought to "purify" the blood by acting as a diuretic (helping the body to get rid of excess fluid) and expectorant (helping clear lungs of mucous), improving circulation, and helping cleanse the liver."

Plant Description:

Red clover is a perennial herb that commonly grows wild in meadows throughout Europe and Asia, and has now been naturalized to grow in North America. The red flowers at the end of the branched stems are usually dried for therapeutic use."

Medicinal Uses and Indication:

"Red clover is a source of many nutrients including calcium, chromium, magnesium, niacin phosphorus, potassium, thiamine, and vitamin C. Red clover is a rich source of isoflavones (chemicals that act like estrogens and are found in many plants.)"

Cancer:

Based on its traditional use for cancer, researchers have begun to study isoflavones from red clover. There is some preliminary evidence that they may stop cancer cells from growing or kill cancer cells in test tubes. But because of the herb's estrogen-like effects, it might also contribute to the growth of some cancers, just as estrogen does. Until further research is done, red clover cannot be recommended to prevent cancer."

Additional information from http:/www.all4naturalhealth.com/red-clover-benefits.html, supports this information. "Red clover is a sweet herb and is considered a blood purifier. It may be used to treat acne, bladder infections, boils, bronchitis, cancer, leukemia, liver disorders, nervous conditions, psoriasis, skin ailments and tumors. It is an excellent blood cleanser."

"Due to its roots running deep into the inner recesses of the earth, red clover is found to be rich in minerals and this fact is obvious from its constituents of caffeic and acids, beta-sitosterol, coumarin, eugenol, flavonoids, salicylic acid, methyl salicylate, calcium, selenium, iron, magnesium, manganese, phosphorous, zinc, molybdenum, beta-carotene and vitamins B, C, and E."

Red Clover and Cancer:

Red clover benefits cancer sufferers, too. The National Cancer Institute has validated the fact that red clover, due to its anti-cancer properties, is effective in combating cancer.

"Traditionally, red clover has been used as a cancer combatant. Modern studies on isoflavones have further shown initial evidence that they may prevent the growth of cancer cells in a lab environment. Hence, it has been postulated that red clover may prevent some forms of cancer, such as endometrial and prostate cancer."

"A note of caution is, however, advised, as red clover mimics the effects of estrogens, and estrogens are sometimes a contributor to cancer. Red clover benefits against cancer can be harnessed externally too. It is frequently used externally in poultice form, as a local application for cancerous growths, and found to be effective."

"Please note that cancer is a serious and multi-factorial disease. It thus needs to be dealt with using a full-spectrum, holistic approach. Using one or two herbs is unlikely to reverse the situation."

The Web site http://www.herbwisdom.com/herb-red-clover.html provides similar information that verifies much of the information shared from the two previously mentioned Web sites.

Notes

Appendix X: Cellular Forte Max3

Appendix X is devoted to the description of a remarkable product named Cellular Forté Max3. I discovered it while exploring the Only Natural Pet Store Web site. I studied the Web site to learn about evidence-based products that were available to help with Oscar's symptoms.

The product's complete name is Integrative Therapeutics Cellular Forté Max3. It is easily found on a search (type in the name of the product in the search box at the top of the page). According to http://www.onlynaturalpet.com, "When our companions are faced with a very serious condition such as immune problems at a cellular level, they need powerful support for their immune systems. Cellular Forte Max3 provides triple strength support to boost natural killer-cell and immune system activity."

"Cells are the structural units of all living things. Dogs and cats have trillions of cells performing all the essential functions of life. Normal, healthy cells are responsible for the beating of the heart, breathing, digesting food, chasing a ball, climbing a tree, wagging a tail and purring. In some cases, however, cells stop functioning or behaving as they should. These cells serve no useful purpose in the body, but may continue to reproduce themselves in a haphazard manner. The body produces it's own immune system cells, including B- and T-cells, dubbed "natural killer-cells" whose job it is to seek and destroy wayward cells. A sick and weakened animal, however, needs extra support for it's immune system to perform this crucial function."

"Triple-powered Cellular Forté Max3 features an exclusive, clinically-studied combination of IP-6 and inositol, maitake D-fraction, and POA cat's claw which are essential for regulating healthy cell development and delivering life-changing results. The patented combination of IP-6 and inositol dramatically increases natural killer-cell activity. Maitake has been shown in clinical research to nutritionally support the growth of healthy cells. POA cat's claw is patented and clinically studied to benefit both the natural and acquired immune systems, plus enhance critical B- and T-cell effectiveness. Together, the ingredients in Cellular Forté Max3 deliver exceptional support for the most critical cells in your immune system."

This product worked remarkably well in combination with the other treatment remedies. I would strongly recommend its use in a treatment plan. The product's triple strength effectiveness was easily observed as I monitored Oscar's condition, and I replaced PhytoPharmica Cellular Forté with Ip-6 & Inositol with this wonderful product. There were five reviews of Cellular Forté Max3 available on www.onlynaturalpet.com, and each emphasized its effectiveness.

Notes

Notes

Notes

CPSIA information can be obtained at www.ICGtesting.com
Printed in the USA
BVOW032358080812

297431BV00001B/2/P